STIGMA

An Ethnography of Mental Illness
and HIV/AIDS in China

STIGMA

An Ethnography of Mental Illness and HIV/AIDS in China

Jinhua Guo
Peking University, China

World Century

Published by

World Century Publishing Corporation
27 Warren Street, Suite 401-402, Hackensack, NJ 07601

Library of Congress Cataloging-in-Publication Data
Names: Guo, Jinhua (Associate professor)
Title: Stigma : an ethnography of mental illness and HIV/AIDS in China / Jinhua Guo (Peking University, China).
Description: New Jersey : World Century, 2016.
Identifiers: LCCN 2015040537 | ISBN 9781938134807 (alk. paper)
Subjects: LCSH: Mental illness--Social aspects--China. | HIV infections--Social aspects--China. | AIDS (Disease)--Social aspects--China.
Classification: LCC RC460 .G86 2016 | DDC 362.19697/9200951--dc23
LC record available at http://lccn.loc.gov/2015040537

British Library Cataloguing-in-Publication Data
A catalogue record for this book is available from the British Library.

In-house Editors: Suraj Kumar/Qi Xiao

Typeset by Stallion Press
Email: enquiries@stallionpress.com

About the Book

Based on two and a half years of fieldwork in China from 2005 to 2007, this book is aimed to examine the cultural genesis and social mechanisms of stigma related to mental illness and HIV/AIDS in China. In Chinese society where concern about human rights is weak, if it is not completely absent, because of the moral common sense of what makes a person, people with mental illness and HIV/AIDS are categorized into the group of non-persons. Non-persons do not experience social acceptance. They are socially excluded. They do not have rights. And thus they are stigmatized and discriminated against. This dangerous cultural form of moral common sense, and the ways families, local communities and state institutions respond to perceived social insecurity — the threat allegedly posed by people who have mental illnesses and HIV/AIDS — mutually shape each other. They work to maintain and strengthen the cruel and injurious stigma associated with mental illness and HIV/AIDS.

In the Chinese context, people with mental illness are considered to be non-persons on account of their mental disabilities; while people with HIV/AIDS are regarded as non-persons because of what they are believed to have done that caused their HIV/AIDS status. I trace how people with mental illness and HIV/AIDS are socially excluded from their existing social relationships and social networks in their local communities. I highlight families as a major site of stigma to describe the micro sociodynamic process of stigmatization in the local context. People with mental illness usually experience a terrible identity transformation: From being a person to being a non-person and, in the extreme case of psychosis, to being a non-human who is rejected and abandoned by the family. People with HIV/AIDS generally experience the reverse transformation: From being a non-human in the family to being a non-person in society.

Through comparison of mental illness and HIV/AIDS, I connect Chinese society and its community-centered social value system to the stigma associated with mental illness and HIV/AIDS. I analyze how discrimination is understood in Chinese daily life and explore the links between disadvantaged groups and the stigmatized. Ultimately this research implies the need to develop human rights-concerned legislation and national policies. It also strongly supports the development of humanitarian ethics-centered professional education and institutional reform in health care systems and public education among the general population in China in order to counteract the catastrophic effect of stigma associated with mental illness and HIV/AIDS and other human conditions.

Jinhua Guo

Contents

Acknowledgments

Without the generous help and consistent support of many people, I would have never been able to complete this work. Arthur and Joan Kleinman are at the top of the list of people to whom I owe a lifetime's gratitude. During the seven years of my studying anthropology at Harvard University (2001–2008), Arthur and Joan guided and cared for me without any reservation. The Chinese saying states that "*yi ri wei shi, zhong sheng wei fu*", meaning that he who teaches you for a day deserves to be respected as your father for a lifetime. I am not sure if I have treated Arthur and Joan as the Chinese saying requires, but they have been taking care of me with all their hearts as if I were one of their children. What Arthur has been giving to me is not just academic training, such as teaching me in the classroom, guiding my reading, giving comments on my works, helping me with my language and even editing my writing, but the long-term care and education to think and act as a responsible scholar who really cares seriously about society and the subjects he is studying. The most valuable lesson I have learned from Arthur is that a medical anthropologist, rather than just using abstract theories to argue about and criticize a variety of unjust human conditions, must always make equal efforts to work with institutions to change and improve these conditions.

I also want to express my gratitude to many professors in the Department of Anthropology at Harvard University. Professors Byron Good and Steve Caton are on my dissertation committee. They have been teaching me, supervising my research and offering me valuable guidance, advice and comments. I would also like to thank Professors James Watson, Theodore C. Bestor, Mary Steedly, Michael Herzfeld and Nur Yalman for letting me sit in their classrooms and listen to their instruction. I am deeply grateful to Marilyn Goodrich (Dr. Kleinman's Faculty Assistant), Sue Hilditch (Wing Assistant of Social Anthropology), Marianne Fritz (Graduate Program Administrator) and Monica Munson (Director of Administration of the Department) for always rescuing me whenever I asked them for help. An extra thanks goes to Marilyn and Marianne for helping me with English language writing style. The Harvard–Yenching Institute sponsored my study at Harvard University. My field research was supported by the Department of Anthropology and by the Michael Crichton Fund for medical anthropology in the Department of Social Medicine, Harvard Medical School. I also received financial support from the Graduate School of Arts and Science at Harvard University. I am grateful to all these institutions.

In China, my fieldwork of two and a half years from 2005 to 2007 would have been impossible without the friendship and hospitality of many medical professionals and other staff members working at the institutions I visited. They are Drs. Du Hui, Yuan Shutian, Zhang Junfeng, Zhong Bao and Zhao Pu in Jian'an City, Hubei Province; Huang Shuanglong, Director of the local health bureau and Dr. Xiao Zhibing in Jiangxia City, Hubei Province; Party Secretary Liu Jianying, Youth League's Secretary Han Jing, Drs. Xu Keyi, Lun Wenhui and Wang Kerong at Ditan Hospital in Beijing; Drs. Zhang Jianbo, Li Qingling, Yang Diao and Yang Chaogui, and Nurse-in-Chief Zhou Xuying and nurses Yang Ling, Liu Yuling, Liu Chunyan and Yang Jia in Dexin City, Yunnan Province. A special thanks goes to hundreds of anonymous patients and their families I met during fieldwork. They educated me through their own life experience and I learned deeply about how they have been struggling to live a moral life in situations featuring social exclusion.

I am also grateful to Gao Qin at Fordham University and Hou Xin at China Youth University for Political Science for introducing me to the relevant institutions and giving me advice on my fieldwork. My fieldwork in Beijing would have been much more difficult without their help. My research also benefited from the advice given by Professors Sun Liping,

Shen Yuan, Guo Yuhua and Jing Jun at Tsinghua University and Ma Mingjie at China Youth Daily. Wu Fei at Peking University and Hu Zongze at Harvard University helped me shape my early thoughts on this research. I also want to thank Lora, Matt, Ahmar and James from Boston University, Fan Wen, Li Tao and Zeng Jing in China for the time we worked together in Dexin.

I owe my sincere apology and gratitude to my parents and Yingran. For the past seven years, on account of my studies I was not able to spend more time with them and take care of them; instead, they always were concerned and worried about me. No one other than Yingran understands what I have been through these years. Her love and resilience always enable me to keep going forward. To her, I owe a promise of a lifetime.

Jinhua Guo

Introduction

Medical anthropology is aimed at exploring meanings in local life world through observing and understanding medical practices and illness experiences in a broader social context. In this research, I focus on stigma associated with mental illness and HIV/AIDS in China and write stigma as part of illness experiences related to mental illness and HIV/AIDS.

There is no doubt that mental illness and HIV/AIDS have caused tragic outcome and unbearable suffering to people who live with the illnesses. Stigma associated with mental illness and HIV/AIDS is a universal social phenomenon across various cultures around the world. In this research, I intend to examine the social genesis, formation and mechanism of stigma related to mental illness and HIV/AIDS in the local context of China.

In current China, stigma constitutes a critical site through which we can observe the radical impact of the profound social transformation toward market economy upon the whole of society: Unbearable social exclusion of various marginalized groups and pervasive feeling of insecurity among the general population. Stigma casts light on usually invisible social suffering and makes it distinct. On one hand, stigma reveals social injustice and social suffering imposed onto marginalized groups by the entire society; on the other hand, stigma demonstrates the pervasive feeling of insecurity in the same society. In today's China, social injustice and suffering have been tolerated, accepted, even legitimatized as if they are the price the country has to pay on its way to a richer and stronger modern nation. In the face of such radical social transformation, the state, to some extent, is sacrificing its legitimacy — social justice — in order to re-legitimatize itself; disadvantaged groups have to sacrifice even the rights to be normal humans in order to survive. The two facts constitute an ironic and painful image in contrast to that built on the far better known flourishing modernization and economic increase.

A society is structured, shaped and maintained by not only social inclusion and solidarity but also social exclusion and isolation. Besides the normal conditions of a society, social suffering provides us another significant angle to look into the society. In this sense, stigma related to diseases, as a part of illness experience both inside and beyond particular culture, is a critical site where anthropologists can observe and understand how society is constituted, how culture is practiced and what really matters in the local world.

In this ethnography of stigma, I try to write in a way that does not create others. Rather than write about the stigmatized as other and about the stigmatizers as another other, I wish to describe the whole situation confronting both the stigmatized and stigmatizers and also my engagement in the local life world through my field work. In so doing, I intend to present a fuller image of stigma and social suffering in China.

Background

Global context

Facing the critical challenges brought by the epidemics of mental illness and HIV/AIDS, many scholars in social science and medicine have come to realize that stigma is as central to the challenge as the diseases (Mann 1987). It has been widely agreed that: stigma does exist; it has exerted profound influence on patients, their families, local communities and even medical professionals and health care institutions; and that stigma has become another barrier in addition to lack of financial support and absence of medical technology to the creation of effective responses to these painful diseases.

Unfortunately, high recognition of stigma on the societal level has not yet led to improved outcome or a more promising future in the battle against stigma. The coexistence of increasing concern and poor understanding has even further marginalized the issue of stigma and constitutes a paradox. As Parker and Aggleton (2003) write, "Issues of stigma, discrimination and denial have been poorly understood and often marginalized within national and international programs and responses" (2003:13). Apparently, stigma associated with diseases has not been paid enough attention in reality as some professionals have claimed, even though none would deny the existence of stigma and its negative influence upon patients and their families. For many medical professionals, stigma remains a secondary issue; the primary task is to find effective treatment. This paradoxical situation indicates that biomedicine is still widely accepted as the single legitimate discourse in responding to the suffering brought about by diseases. Hence, the cure of disease is considered the ultimate way to remove stigma. That is to say, stigma will disappear once the disease is cured.

More paradoxical are the coexistence of high recognition of stigma and high level of stigmatization and that of ongoing stigmatization and increasing voices calling for anti-stigmatization. Medical professionals often tend to attribute stigma to people's not possessing the correct knowledge of the diseases; among the general population there is a common belief that the dramatic social transformation result in lack of sympathy for sufferers. It is neither surprising nor confusing that stigmatization continues if stigmatizing and destigmatizing positions are held by different persons; but it is noteworthy that the two voices may come from the same subjects who say one thing and do another. Either the same subject has not noticed the disjuncture between the two voices, or the awareness of such a disjuncture does not make any difference to the person in his/her action. In other words, such a disjuncture does not seem to be a disjuncture for a single person. This paradoxical fact suggests that stigma is maintained by some meaningful ambiguity spreading over local knowledge. In this sense, the paradox and ambiguity appeared in anti-stigma campaign may provide an angle to look into stigma.

Chinese context

According to data from China's Ministry of Health, 16 million people are suffering from various mental illnesses, of which schizophrenia is at the top of the list with 6 million people afflicted; each year China has 100,000 more patients diagnosed with mental illnesses. However, the number of all available sickbeds for mental illness is less than 150,000 by the end of 2006, including the sickbeds in mental hospitals and psychiatry sections in general hospitals. There is a huge gap between the demand for medical care and the available care resources. Less than 10% of mentally ill persons are receiving treatment (Zhang 2006).

In addition to the shortage of mental health care resources, stigma associated with mental illness forms another obstruction both for patients to seek effective help and for mental health care system to deliver the service. Stigma related to mental illness makes the current limited mental health care resources even unavailable for those who need help; hence, people with mental illness often live in worse condition than that caused by illness itself. In China, among the reports related to mental illness that can be read about in public media, people with psychosis play a leading role with pejorative overtones and violent events, in which either mentally ill persons attacked or killed others or they were killed. People with mental illness are described retarded or dangerous.

The first HIV case in China was discovered in 1985. By the end of the 1980s, the first wave of infection stormed Yunnan, a province located in the south of China, bordering Southern Asian countries such as Thailand and Burma. Since the middle 1990s, China has entered a rapidly increasing phase of HIV/AIDS infection. In 2003, data released by China's Ministry of Health indicated that the number of people who have been infected was estimated at 1,000,000, of which 850,000 are alive; 95% of HIV/AIDS patients have not been located, most of them do not know they are infected; blood transfusion, drug abuse and commercial sex have been recognized as major infection routes (A Joint Assessment of HIV/AIDS Prevention, Treatment and Care in China, 2003). The difference in infection routes has exerted significant influence on stigma associated with HIV/AIDS patients. Drug users, commercial sex workers and gay men generally hesitate to seek help because of strongly perceived stigma and discrimination against themselves; while people who contract AIDS during blood selling and blood transfusion often consider themselves innocent victims. They are likely to speak out in public and seek compensation and medical help. Hence, their HIV/AIDS identity is more easily exposed in the society. In this sense, these innocent victims often have a more painful life experience than other patients. Most of these patients are from the poorest rural areas of China, especially in Henan province. Research showed that stigma remained even after villagers correctly possessed medical knowledge of HIV/AIDS, and that stigma related to HIV/AIDS often spread from patients to their families, even the village (Gao *et al.* 2004). Public media reported that many families with HIV/AIDS members were either locked up behind walls constructed by villagers or kicked out of the village; their children were forced to quit school; in some cases, the entire village was stigmatized and isolated, people from other villages refused to visit or do business with the village (Tang *et al.* 2004; Wang 2008). Stigma related to HIV/AIDS also exists in health care institutions in China. General hospitals often refuse to receive people who contracted HIV/AIDS (Li *et al.* 2007; Wang and Zhang 2006). Among the medical professionals working with mental illness and HIV/AIDS, there is a noticeable disparity between attitude and practices (Peng *et al.* 2006).

It is noteworthy that the Chinese government's initial responses to HIV/AIDS epidemic to some extent maintained and strengthened stigma related to the illness. By classifying patients into several subgroups in terms of infection routes (blood selling, blood transfusing, drug abuse and commercial sex), the Chinese government divided HIV/AIDS patients into different groups at different levels of social status. In the beginning, the state only provided free HIV test and medication to "innocent patients" who were infected during blood selling, and later they changed the policy to cover the entire HIV/AIDS group. In a sense, stigma has been legitimatized by the state's policy, even though the same government is also supporting anti-stigma campaigns. In fact, the government's differentiation of HIV/AIDS patients is a distinct embodiment of stigma rooted in Chinese society.

In fighting HIV/AIDS epidemic, the government at all levels in China often apply the strategy of scaring people away from contracting the illness, which further strengthens stigma related to HIV/AIDS among the general population. In a context featuring fear, both HIV/AIDS patients and others tend to abuse HIV/AIDS related stigma. Public reports showed that, in some cities, thieves claimed that they had HIV/AIDS when they were caught by the police, or intentionally have themselves infected, in order to escape from the law. Their confidence was based on two facts: the police were afraid of HIV/AIDS patients too; the justice system was not ready yet for the new situation brought about by HIV/AIDS and did not have the institutional arrangements for criminals with HIV/AIDS status (Feng and Li 2007). In some places, HIV/AIDS patients were said to have been hired to do debt collecting because none dare to turn down people with HIV/AIDS. There were also rumors going on in several cities (Beijing, Shanghai, Tianjing and Guangzhou in 2002; Shanghai, Nanjing and Hangzhou in 2005) from time to time during the period of 2001–2005, saying HIV/AIDS patients were trying to attack other people with infected syringes to have more and more people infected with HIV in order to revenge the society. All of these rumors have never been confirmed, yet showed the pervasive "moral panic and trust crisis" of the Chinese society in the face of HIV/AIDS epidemic (Jing 2006).

Research Design

The majority of the previous studies concerning stigma have been focusing on the stigmatized while the image of the stigmatizer has been either absent, invisible or blurred. Few studies have provided detailed anthropological analysis on the social genesis and the operating and maintaining mechanism of stigma. I propose to reconsider stigma associated with mental illness and HIV/AIDS in the context of local life worlds shaped by everyday practices in the face of the threat and danger posed by the two diseases. My ethnography is aimed to examine stigma in the context of local life by describing experiences of stigma from both the side of the stigmatized and the stigmatizers. This research is based on my understanding of illness as a critical situation emerging within the local life world. Stigma, I conceive, is a daily practical response to this critical situation.

In August of 2003, I conducted one-month of preliminary field research in Jian'an and Jiangxia cities of Hubei province in China. This preliminary research was a great help for me to adjust my research plan according to what I had encountered in the field. Originally I planned to conduct field research in three sites, one big city, one small town and one village. After preliminary research, I realized that it was going to be difficult for me to focus simultaneously on two objects (mental illness and HIV/AIDS) at each of the three sites. Therefore I decided to make a change to my original plan: I set up two sites (one urban and one rural) for both mental illness and HIV/AIDS, respectively. Two types of research methods were used in my fieldwork: short-time interviews and long-term participant observation. Local hospitals treating the two illnesses were the major places where I got involved and started my research in communities; doing volunteer work in local clinics was the main method I used to get familiar with my research subjects and conduct interviews and further long-term participant observation. My field research ethnography started in early 2005 and ended in June 2007.

Overall, I conducted field research in the following four phases:

1. From January to August of 2005, I worked on mental illness in my hometown, Jian'an, which is located in central China. My major concern was the stigma associated with mental illness in urban context. The Psychiatric Clinic of the Third People's Hospital in Jian'an was where I conducted my research. My research included interviews with 10 patients with mental illness, four medical professionals and four patients' families.

2. From September 2005 to January 2006, I conducted research in Jiangxia city, also in Hubei, on mental illness. I focused on stigma related to mental illness in rural area and how it compares to stigma in urban areas like Jian'an. My research site was Jiangxia Mental Hospital. I interviewed 15 patients with mental illness, five medical professionals and five patients' families.

3. From March to December in 2006, I moved to Beijing and did fieldwork on HIV/AIDS. My focus was stigma associated with HIV/AIDS among a gay men's group in Beijing and how it compares to stigma associated with mental illness. I met hundreds of HIV/AIDS patients at AIDS Care Center in the Fourth People's Hospital, conducted 30 detailed interviews with patients and 10 with medical professionals and 10 with patients' families. It was a valuable experience of long-term participant observation. While doing volunteer work I conducted field research at this Center. My volunteer work helped me get very familiar with doctors, nurses, patients and their families and conduct deep participant observation.

4. In 2007, from January to June, I went to Dexin in Yunnan Province in South China and conducted field research on the second phase of my HIV/AIDS project. This research opportunity came from my good relationship with AIDS Care Center in Beijing. In the last month of my research in Beijing, the director of the STD Department of the Fourth People's Hospital asked me to help them conduct a HIV/AIDS related medical project among drug users in Yunnan, which was exactly the research site I was looking for at the time. Moreover, the place in Yunnan was a Bai ethnic minority rural area. Therefore I accepted this invitation without any hesitation and soon left for Yunnan. In Yunnan, my research objectives were: Stigma associated with HIV/AIDS among drug users in Bai ethnic minority area, how it compares to stigma among gay men's groups in Beijing, and how it compares to stigma associated with mental illness.

During all my field research, my major concerns were: (1) How do patients, patients' families, medical professionals and local communities view and understand the two illnesses? (2) How do they live or work with the two illnesses respectively? (3) How do patients, patients' families, medical professionals and the local community feel and think about the problem of stigma associated with the two illnesses? (4) What are (national and local) governments' policies and their practices under these policies when it comes to the two illnesses? (5) What do these illnesses mean to patients, patients' families, medical professionals and local communities? (6) What are the differences in stigma between urban and rural areas? (7) What are the differences in stigma associated with mental illness and stigma associated with HIV/AIDS?

All names (including cities, hospitals, institutions and individual informants) and identifying details in all of those cases present in this research have been changed. This is to ensure confidentiality and protect the anonymity of all informants involved.

Chapter One

Theoretical reviews and critiques

Psychological and Social Psychological Models

Psychology has played a prominent role in studies of stigma. Goffman has been widely referred to as the first to conceptualize stigma within social psychology and sociology. In his classic book — *Stigma: Notes on the Management of Spoiled Identity* (Goffman 1963) — Goffman defines stigma as "an attribute that is deeply discrediting" (1986:3), which causes a spoiled identity and results in the reduction of a person (or group) "from a whole and usual person to a tainted, discounted one" (1986:3). In his view, discrediting attributes, such as mental illness, physical deformity, and socially deviant behavior, spoil the identity of subjects and make them "not quite human" (1986:5). Goffman's view has shaped the way later scholars understand stigma, "stigma comes to be seen as something in the person stigmatized, rather than as a designation that others attach to that individual" (Link and Phelan, 2001). In the same book, Goffman primarily focuses on how normal persons respond to the stigmatized and how the stigmatized manage self-presentation in daily life in order to cope with stigmatizing situations. Without considering broader social context, Goffman limits stigmatization in a generalized individual perspective of social interaction. The process from discrediting attribute to spoiled identity and onto subsequent consequence — how a discrediting attribute, as part of personal characteristics, spoils the whole identity — is far beyond his interpretation of the discrepancy between social expectation and reality, or normality and deviation. The questions left by Goffman are what makes a discrediting attribute in a society and how such a discrediting attribute lead to a spoiled identity.

Jones *et al.* (1984) reformulate a social psychological view of stigma. They substitute mark for Goffman's concept of discrediting attribute. "Mark is our generic term for perceived or inferred conditions of deviation from a prototype or norm that might initiate the stigmatizing process" and a discrediting mark makes a person markable (1984:8). Jones *et al.* also identify six dimensions of stigma: concealability, course, disruptiveness, aesthetics, origin, and peril. Yet the real advance they make, in my view, lies in that they relocate stigma in the context of social interaction and relationship. "The marked person may or may not be stigmatized. To mark a person implies that the deviant condition has been noticed and recognized as a problem in the interaction or relationship. To stigmatize a person generally carries a further implication that the mark has been linked by an attribution process to dispositions that discredit the bearer, i.e., that spoil his identity" (1984:8). In their view, it is "impression engulfment" accumulated in social interaction that drives the marking process into "the more devastating realm of stigma" (1984:8). In this sense, Jones *et al.* bridge the gap between "discrediting attribute" and "spoiled identity" with a process of impression engulfment. But, in actual world, stigma does not always result from impression engulfment formed in face to face interaction. For example, public stigma exists and remains even without face-to-face interaction between normal person and deviant individual; instead, many people do not have any personal contact with mentally ill persons or HIV/AIDS patients. For these people, such deviant individuals exist as an imagined community living somewhere, but stigma exists and remains. In this sense, social interaction is not a necessary factor for the formation of stigma. In addition, Jones *et al.* try to generalize stigmatization. They write, "Such relationships [of stigmatization] are neither rare nor esoteric. We have all participated in them, either as the deviant or as the normal partner" (1984:1). It is insightful to point out that stigma is a common social phenomenon, in which everyone is possibly involved, because everyone has experience of being marked and marking others. However, as they say, mark does not always make stigma. Jones *et al.* seem to confuse mark with stigma. This confusion reduces stigma into mark, which apparently does not do justice to those who have the most painful experience of being stigmatized. In a sense, Jones *et al.* generalize the meaning of suffering. Being stigmatized is not just about being seen or treated differently but unfairly and even inhumanly in many cases. The way Jones *et al.* generalize stigma obscures the boundary between suffering caused by mark and suffering caused by stigma.

Alonzo and Reynolds (1995) suggest that stigma is a social constructive/interactive phenomenon, "not static but emergent and something that can be said to be undergone and experienced" (1995:313), and it "is expansive, pervading all corners of one's life space and identity" (1995:313). Alonzo and Reynolds define the stigmatized as "a category of people who are pejoratively regarded by the broader society and who are devalued, shunned or otherwise lessened in their life chances and in access to the humanizing benefit of free and unfettered social intercourse" (1995:304). Based on Goffman's definition of spoiled identity and Jones *et al.*'s multidimensional concept of stigma, Alonzo and Reynolds list the components of stigma related to HIV/AIDS: Deviant behavior, individual responsibility, immorality in terms of religious belief, contagious and threatening realities, undesirable and unaesthetic death, and misunderstanding by lay community and negative view from health care providers. They point out that stigma has usually not been considered as changing and emerging over the course of a single illness, even though it has been generally recognized that the nature of stigma varies across illnesses (1995:313). Hence, they raise a concept of stigma trajectory, describe how persons with HIV/AIDS experience a stigma trajectory over four phases of the disease course (at risk, diagnosis, latent and manifest state), and demonstrate how stigmatizing experiences are affected by changes in the biophysical dimensions of HIV/AIDS. Alonzo and Reynolds' stigma dynamics is based on disease dynamics; however, they neglect the involvement of broader social context in the process of stigmatization.

Link and Phelan (2001) conceptualize stigma in the perspective of social cognition. They bring in the concept of power and point out that stigma is entirely dependent on social, economic and political power. They identify five interrelated components (labeling, stereotyping, separation, status loss and discrimination) and propose that stigma comes into being when the five components co-occur in a power situation. Link and Phelan define power (social, cultural, economic and political) as a crucial factor that determines whether or not labeling, stereotyping and cognitive separation result in serious discriminatory consequences. However, Link and Phelan seem to understand power as an existing structure and pay no attention to the fact that power can also be reproduced any time. It may be true that lower-power groups have no chance to stigmatize higher-power groups in some situations, but that does not mean that stigmatization will not happen in higher-power group. Link and Phelan's understanding of the contribution of power difference to stigmatization is limited by their static view of power. Stigma is not just a result of power difference but also a source of power difference.

Stigma studies in social history

Besides social psychology oriented studies, social history is another important field where stigma theory has been written. Gussow (1989) explores the transformation of stigma related to leprosy in the historical context, which makes a fundamental difference to social psychology's writings about stigma. Gussow writes the history of leprosy stigma in a changing context framed by colonial encounter, religious thoughts, popular beliefs, and national policies. In his book, the history of leprosy stigma is related to a human history of relating physical unsightliness and disgustingness to backwardness and moral uncleanness in the soul, and a history of stigmatizing particular race (Yellow peril) and territory (oriental leprosy). As leprosy changed from a hereditary disease to a germ based disease, its implication altered from a punishment on a morally unclean race to a serious threat perceived by normal population; at the same time, the role of people with leprosy transformed from the bearer of stigma to the carrier of stigma, and the meaning of space also transferred from the guarantee of safety to a container of danger.

Watts (1997) attributes stigmatization of epidemics to western construct and the expansion of imperialism. Taking leprosy for example, Watts points out that there is a big difference in the attitude toward leprosy between colonists and colonials. In his view, the discovery of other cultures does not constitute a reflection of colonists on their own culture and the knowledge they assumed; instead, cultural difference becomes evidence of the distinction between the civilized and the barbarous. "Central to the thinking of western workers in leprosy before 1980 was the idea that civilized people everywhere shunned lepers; any cultural group which didn't behave in this way was barbarous or at least semi-civilized." In this sense, stigma is the evidence of being the civilized while the barbarous do not stigmatize. Watts further notes that this also applies to rural medieval Europe, which even suggests that stigma is nothing but a product of power relationships. Yet Watts seems to believes that stigma related to leprosy is absent in some cultures simply because of no fear for the disease. It may be true in the case of leprosy, but he apparently turn to use culture rather than power relationships to define stigma. Moreover, not all power relationships are brought by the colonists into the colonies; power relationships have also existed in many colonized cultures before the colonists invaded.

Sociological perspectives

More recently, Parker and Aggleton (2003) argue that stigma studies are facing serious conceptual limitation and even no definition while dictionary definitions and common sense definitions are widely used without serious reflection. Most stigma studies, in their opinion, are simple reproductions featuring a social cognitive focus and individualistic emphasis started and encouraged by Goffman. These studies seek to understand stigma in highly emotional terms and focus on stigmatizing attitude that is, as generally assumed, caused by misunderstandings, misinformation, beliefs and attitudes of perceived stigmatizers. Parker and Aggleton believe that these problems have misled and reduced current intervention programs on stigma into giving correct information, increasing tolerance, empathy and altruism, reducing anxiety and fear, increasing contact and helping the stigmatized acquire coping skills. To move beyond these limitations, Parker and Aggleton bring in a sociological emphasis on the structural dimension of discrimination, which was raised by Marshall (1998), and reframe stigmatization and discrimination as "social process that can only be understood in relation to broader notions of power and domination" (2003:16). Parker and Aggleton try to relocate stigma in a context framed by culture, power, and difference. They recognize that "stigma plays a key role in producing and reproducing relations of power and control" (2003:16) and focus on "how stigma is used by individuals, communities and the state to produce and reproduce social inequality" (2003:17). In the end, they raise the concept of political economy of stigmatization and social exclusion. Parker and Aggleton improve Link and Phelan's definition of power by acknowledging power/domination as a product of stigmatization. They primarily focus on the role played by stigmatization in producing and reproducing power relationships and social inequality. In other words, they are more interested in social, cultural and political appropriation of stigma than stigmatization itself. Parker and Aggleton ground stigma in broader social context, which is a promising direction. However, they may study stigma but divert to another and end up in academic appropriation of stigma: the real object of stigma studies is likely to melt away in the context of culture, power and difference and to be replaced by the discourses of power and domination. In that case, stigma turns out to be a newfound raw material for the reproduction of academic discourse on power. The new direction showed by Park and Aggleton is promising, but it will not help much if we jump onto the topic of power without hesitation and without reflection its limits.

Anthropological views on stigma

Anthropological efforts of exploring the meaning of stigma can be traced to Mary Douglas's analysis (1994) of minority risks. Douglas defines stigma as the practices of "moralizing danger" (persecution of moral deviants in the name of dangers) — a strategy for exclusion and rejection. She focuses on the condition in which the stigmatized are living, intends to detach stigma from the stigmatized themselves and relocates it in broader social context. Taking witchcraft and leprosy for example, Douglas sorts out the mechanism of social rejection: libel, imputation of immorality, and accusation of causing damage.

Medical anthropologist Arthur Kleinman calls for attention to the cultural meaning behind stigma associated with mental illness and other diseases in his *The Illness Narratives* (1988). To quote his words, "a disfiguring deformity and the bizarre actions of florid mental illness stigmatize because they break cultural conventions about what is acceptable appearance and behavior, while invoking other cultural categories of what is ugly, feared, alien or inhuman" (1988:159). He points out that "stigma helps to define the social identity of the group" (1988:159) and acceptance of the stigmatized identity makes patients feel shame in their interactions with families and health professionals. For stigma associated with mental illness in China, he writes, "The stigma of mental illness is so powerful that it attaches not only to the seriously mentally ill but also to their families" (1988:160). Kleinman suggests that there is a difference in the social genesis of stigma between China and the United Sates. In his view, in Chinese context, the collapse of social network caused by mental illness is the main reason that people with mental illness are stigmatized; in the United Sates, the reason is the socially perceived individual incapacity caused by mental illness. In his *What Really Matters* (2006), he points out that, during the Cultural Revolution in China, people outside of the "red" sectors were stigmatized as class enemies because of their "black" family background, such as businessmen, homeowners, landowners, liberal intellectuals, and members of other political parties. Stigma caused "restriction of living conditions" and restriction on the opportunities to build one's own life and career as one wants (2006:86).

Farmer (1992) analyzes the accusation and blame associated with AIDS epidemic in Haiti and proposes that sickness is the result of structural violence and behind the discrimination against people who have HIV/AIDS is a strong stigma against marginal groups. His research reminds us of the stigma against outsiders, immigrants, and inside members who have contact with outsiders in the face of infectious diseases, as Gussow mentions in his study of leprosy. Both Gussow and Farmer reveal that stigma has much to do with whom to blame and accuse in the face of threat and danger. By defining sickness as a result of structural violence, Farmer suggested that stigma related to the sickness is also caused by structural violence. Based on research in Brazil, Abadia-Barrero and Castro (2006) found that "structural violence in the forms of poverty, racism, and inequalities in social status, gender, and age fuels children's experiences of stigma", they proposed "structural violence as the framework to study stigma" (2005:1219). Castro and Farmer (2005) stated that the current definition of stigma has not been "grounded in a broader biosocial understanding" and is "often desocialized — decontextualized from larger social processes that are both historically rooted and linked to persons and processes that are not visible to the survey researcher" (2005: 53). They proposed "structural violence as a conceptual framework for understanding AIDS-related stigma" (2005:54). Fassin (2007) also depicted AIDS patients' illness experience in the historical and political context featuring social inequality. Biehl (2005) described people with mental illness and HIV/AIDS in Brazil who were regarded as ex-humans living in a zone of social abandonment.

Based on the concepts of local world and illness experience developed in Kleinman's research, Yang *et al.* (2007) identify stigma as a moral experience by which to understand both the stigmatized and stigmatizers. They state that "stigma exerts its core effects by threatening the loss or diminution of what is most at stake, or by actually diminishing or destroying that lived value." They further bring in the Chinese concept of "face" to highlight the moral dimensions of stigma. Through their efforts, stigma has been relocated in the Chinese local life world and can be examined in the local context shaped by cultural meanings and local moral practices.

The Myths of Stigma in China

In China, stigma did not attract much public attention until the Chinese government defined HIV/AIDS epidemic as a life and death issue to the state. That is to say, it was HIV/AIDS epidemic that forces the country finally to start paying attention to and considering about the issue of stigma. Yet only stigma related to HIV/AIDS has been concerned so far. As HIV/AIDS stigma has been increasingly recognized, both mass media and academic discourses tend to attribute stigma to traditional cultural construction, lack of disease knowledge, and lack of sympathy due to the dramatic social transformation.

1. Cultural construction

It has been widely assumed that the Chinese culture features abstinence, family values, and hesitating about speaking of sex. Many scholars believe these factors are the main sources of stigma related to HIV/AIDS since the disease is still linked to sexual deviance among the general population in China (Shi 2004; Chen *et al.* 2004; Li *et al.* 2005; Cao *et al.* 2005; Liu 2005). In their opinion, the Chinese people generally assumed that only immoral behavior causes HIV/AIDS infection, even though a great number of people contracted HIV/AIDS through drug abuse and blood selling in China; hence, stigmatizing sexual deviance is the source of stigma associated with HIV/AIDS, which means stigma is a result of cultural construction. However, this point of view often stopped here as an explanation of stigma's cultural genesis and could not go further to make a point about how to contribute to anti-stigma campaign. Although many scholars agreed that discrimination against sexual deviance is the source of stigma related to HIV/AIDS, none had questioned the pervasive negative attitude toward sexual deviance in the Chinese society. They either endorsed this attitude or would not take the risk to question it because they would be considered morally incorrect to do so. Therefore, this explanation often went nowhere but turned to seek help from other explanations.

Research conducted in Yi minority area was a typical example (Hou *et al.* 2004; Jiarimuji 2007). Researchers claimed that neither the idea of sexual deviance nor the negative attitude toward sexual deviance existed in Yi culture, which led to the absence of stigma associated with HIV/AIDS in Yi ethnic group. Considering the fact that drug abuse and lack of knowledge of HIV/AIDS were both common in that area, researchers sighed that, without stigma related to HIV/AIDS, this epidemic was going to make this group suffer more. Research of this kind suggests that Chinese scholars often have mixed feeling about cultural conventions with respect to HIV/AIDS stigma. They acknowledged the link between cultural conventions and stigma, but they hardly seriously take cultural conventions as something problematic; moreover, they even consider stigma as an effective measure to prevent the spread of HIV/AIDS epidemic, even though they were criticizing stigma at the same time.

In addition, culture and practice are two mutually constituted fields. Cultural conventions have the power to shape practice, but practice has never been a mirror representation of cultural conventions. The interaction between culture and practice is missed in this cultural explanation with respect to stigma related to HIV/AIDS in China.

2. Lack of correct knowledge of diseases

Around the world, many medical professionals and NGO workers who are managing epidemic prevention and anti-stigma programs have endorsed the view that stigma results from lack of correct knowledge of the disease. That is to say, educating people about the diseases is going to change their behavior and remove stigma related to the disease. China is not an exception (Wang *et al.* 2002; Wang and Zhang 2006). This theory assumes that people simply act on the idea of what is right or wrong in a scientific sense once they get to know it. Such a view is a product of the dominant ideological belief in science: knowledge and technology are the final solutions to any problem even social problems. Yet it has completely neglected or denied the significance of emotions and social values in the formation of stigma. Based on this point of view, correct knowledge is as easy a solution to stigma as medicine to disease. However, research conducted in Africa and Asia shows that anti-stigma campaigns featuring giving correct knowledge and changing behavior have not worked successfully as were assumed. There is a disparity between attitude and behavior; acquiring correct knowledge does not necessarily lead to the expected change in behavior.

In China, HIV/AIDS epidemic education is generally implemented in the form of political propaganda, in which scare tactics are often applied in order to scare people away from contracting HIV/AIDS. In so doing, education does not remove stigma; rather, it create, maintain and strengthen stigma because what people learn from these education programs is nothing other than how dangerous these diseases can be. Even if people are given full and correct knowledge about the disease, they hardly learn the knowledge the way they are supposed to. There is always disparity between giving and receiving information during this process, especially when people perceive risk, dangerousness engulfs all the other parts about the disease.

3. Moral degeneration

This explanation that stigma is a result of moral degeneration sounds very attractive and reasonable, especially in current Chinese society where the profound ongoing economic reform is assumed to have altered social values in the society. People often complain that traditional cultural conventions and social values have collapsed, and that radical social transformation has produced less social sympathy and more self-interested behavior in today's China. The pervasive feeling of insecurity has convinced not only general public but also many scholars that lack of sympathy produced by the social transformation toward the market economy is the main source of increasing social injustice, including stigma. Although most of the Chinese people appreciate the improvement in their lives, at the same time they believe that something valued, such as people's conscience, virtue, and even human nature, in the past have been changed or lost. Considering the broader social context featuring radical social change in China, it is understandable to link stigma to lack of sympathy. However, stigma and other social suffering did not start with the initiation of economic reform; rather, it has a long history in the society and has been related to psychical disability, social deviance, political identity, family background, etc.

In addition, it is ironic to state that people stigmatize because they are morally degenerate and simply have no sympathy for the sufferers, giving the fact that the stigmatized are often considered morally defective too and deserving being stigmatized. In this sense, people who support this view seem to play another moral judge besides stigmatizers who morally judge the stigmatized. While washing out the stigmatized' moral blemish, they attach the same label to others whom they consider are stigmatizers and pick themselves out of the issue of stigma. Such a view can easily lead to create stigmatizers as another other in addition to the stigmatized and reduced stigma into a problem only related to those who have no sympathy. This approach copies the logic and mechanism of stigma and reproduces stigma.

Pre-Research Thoughts

Stigma is neither a problem of the stigmatized, nor a problem of stigmatizers, but a problem of "us", a problem of the entire society. It is a totalizing social phenomenon constituted, shaped, maintained and developed by the joint forces of institutional structure, cultural construction and daily practice in the local life world.

Let me summary my major points:

1. Stigma is a universal human experience present in every society. In the case of mental illness and HIV/AIDS, stigma, as part of illness experience, is shaped by emotions and social values based on moral common

sense in the local world. It is related to the local knowledge regarding how to understand, categorize, and respond to danger and threat in daily life.

2. Stigma has strong moral meanings. It is the embodiment of daily practices of local moral common sense. It refers to how a person comes to be a person and when a person can lose his/her personhood and become a non-person and even non-human. The condition that a person can be stigmatized is that he/she is reduced into a non-person, and even non-human, which is the very reason that the stigmatized can be disregarded, shunned, teased, and abused as a being without personhood or dignity. Therefore, for the stigmatizer, stigmatization means to do justice to non-persons or non-humans. Ignoring or treating the stigmatized inhumanly is considered a normal and moral statement about one's own moral stance. People are stigmatized because they have been deprived of the right to be a person or human. Losing personhood or human identity is not the consequence of stigmatization, but a condition of stigmatization. Therefore, the key to understand stigma is to explore in what situations people are reduced into non-persons or non-humans.

3. Stigma is carried by the stigmatized rather than fixed on them, which renders stigma communicable and reproducible in both space and time. This has been demonstrated by the fact that not only individuals, but also their families, neighborhoods, local communities, medical professionals, health care institutions, and even the whole country (for instance, "yellow fever" in history and SARS in China in 2003) could be stigmatized. Furthermore, the concept of "high-risk group" plays a crucial part in the practice of stigmatization. Especially when the stigmatized are not visible in public, high-risk groups become the main carriers of stigma, even if they do not have the disease. Defining and locating high-risk groups became one of the major tasks in today's epidemiology and public health. The logic and process of identifying high-risk groups reveals who is most likely to be the target of stigmatization. For example, in China, it has been officially taken for granted that migrant rural workers working in urban areas play a major part in the spreading of HIV/AIDS epidemic, many reports also considered migrant workers as one of the high-risk groups with respect to HIV/AIDS epidemic (Chinese Ministry of Health and UNAIDS 2003; National Intelligence Council 2002; Anderson *et al.*

2003). The reason is that migrant workers are assumed to have engaged in more casual sex than other people. However, research (Hesketh *et al.* 2006) conducted in Hangzhou of eastern China showed that "at present HIV is probably not spreading in the internal migrant population in eastern China" and "the tendency to migrate with partners makes migrants relatively low risk for engaging in casual sex" (Hesketh *et al.* 2006:11).

4. Stigma is also reproducible in the dimension of time. In the case of stigma associated with mental illness and HIV/AIDS, it seems that it is the disease that creates stigma. It is not, however, from the first day humans had mental illness and HIV/AIDS that stigma started up. There is a long history that people have been stigmatized because of various health problems, such as leprosy, cancer, diabetes, disability, mental illness, and HIV/AIDS. There is also a history in which people without any physical or mental abnormality or incapacity have been stigmatized because of their social identity, including race, gender, sexual orientation, religion, social class, and political thoughts. In this sense, mental illness and HIV/AIDS are nothing but new vehicles for stigma; people who have mental illness and HIV/AIDS become the new carriers of stigma. In the Chinese context, since the Chinese Communist Party took over the regime in 1949, endless political campaigns have created many objects of stigmatization in the society, such as class enemies, backward people, and rightists. People were stigmatized because of their family background, political ideology and even life style. Since the late 1980s, rural workers and urban unemployed workers have been categorized as dangerous groups which pose a threat to the entire society. Over all these years, the carriers of stigma have changed from political dissidents to the poor population, which is considered a threat to societal security and a high-risk group in dealing with HIV/AIDS epidemic.

5. Stigmatization has been legitimatized, maintained, and strengthened by governmental policies, institutions and their routine practices. Government often utilizes stigmatization as a necessary and effective measure of social control in the face of social crisis and public health crisis.

Chapter Two

Ethnography of stigma associated with mental illness

I started to do my field research in Jian'an of Hubei province, my hometown located in the central part of China, since the end of 2004. I still remember the day I arrived home. After I settled down, my father asked me about my research topic, I told him it is related to mental illness and HIV/AIDS. My father looked at me for a while, and then said, "Why don't you find yourself a decent research topic other than that?" My mother seemed nervous, saying, "We know nothing about your research, but you should make sure to take care of yourself no matter what you are dealing with. We are just worrying about you." Yes, they just worry about me and I know that. From that moment, however, I began to have my own personal experience of what stigma is like in Chinese local life world and came to feel how the stigmatized feel in their daily lives.

At the moment, I did not feel it right to educate my father about what mental illness or HIV/AIDS is, what stigma is, why this research is meaningful in order to defend my research against his view of a "decent" research. It is not because this time the one in front of me is my father whom I am not supposed to educate with respect to Chinese cultural norms, but because stigmatization, rather than being based in the generally alleged ignorance about these illnesses or the increasing social indifference to minority's suffering in today's China, is a seemingly natural human response to danger and threat.

Unlike the pathology of disease in medicine, illness experience is full of judgments concerning emotional and value issues. It is not a choice made based on the scientific sense of right or wrong. Stigma associated with diseases is part of illness experience because it shows how people feel about these diseases in their daily lives. What stigma is about has much to do with what illness means for people living in their local life worlds. People worry out of concern for themselves and others, and stigma results from who and what people worry about. In this sense, stigma sheds a light on the boundary of human concern and worry.

Meanwhile, my parents' reaction to my research made me reconsider the way stigma associated with the two diseases has been approached by researches so far, for whom patients' suffering resulting from the way they are treated locally remains as a major subject. I came to realize that there is need to look into stigma from the perspective of stigmatizers, which, I believe, is significant and necessary for a full understanding of stigma. Why do stigmatizers stigmatize? Simply attributing stigma to either the ignorance or bias of the stigmatizers or the vulnerability of the stigmatized does not do justice to this issue. I argue that stigma should be examined in local contexts featuring the interpersonal experience of illness, and therefore the moral relationships between stigmatizers and the stigmatized.

Jian'an City, Hubei Province

Before I develop this issue ethnographically, I need first to situate my research site in its local contexts: geographic, cultural, socioeconomic, and professional. Hubei province is located in the central part of China. The name Hubei means "north of the lake", referring to Hubei's position north of Dongting Lake. The capital of Hubei is Wuhan, a large industrial city. Hubei borders Henan to the north, Anhui to the east, Jiangxi to the southeast, Hunan to the south, Chongqing to the west and Shaanxi to the northwest. The world famous Three Gorges Dam is located in Yichang city in western Hubei. The Jianghan Plain takes up most of central and eastern Hubei, while the west and the peripheries are full of mountains, of which Wudang Mountain has been known as the cradle of Chinese Taoism. The Yangtze River enters Hubei from the west; thousands of lakes dot the landscape.

Hubei is one of the agricultural centers of China, often called the Land of Fish and Rice. The chief agricultural products include cotton, rice, wheat and tea, while major industries include automobiles, metallurgy, machinery, power generation and textiles. Hubei's economy ranks 12th in China among its 23 provinces, five autonomous regions, and four government-controlled municipalities, meaning that it is not as rich as the eastern provinces or as poor as the western ones. The population of Hubei province was 60 million as of the end of 2005, of which 25 million were registered as urban population. Han is the dominant ethnic group in Hubei, more than 57 million. People in Hubei speak Southwestern Mandarin, a dialect group that encompasses most of southwestern China.

Hubei is divided into 13 prefecture-level divisions, three directly administered county-level cities and one directly administered county-level forestry area. Jian'an is one of those thirteen prefecture-level cities. Jian'an is so named as in ancient times it was the gate of the State of Jing. Jian'an is four hours from Wuhan by bus, and three hours by train. It is surrounded by hills. The economy consists mainly of agriculture and manufacturing. The most important industry is petroleum refining. The Jian'an Branch of Sinopec is a major producer of oil products in central China, refining crude oil extracted from the Nanyang Oilfield in Henan Province and the Jianghan Oilfield in Hubei Province. Other important industries include power generation, the production of agricultural chemicals and cement, and beer making.

The population of Jian'an is approximately 2,984,000. The urban area of Jian'an City has a population of about 350,000. Jian'an City has 546 health care institutions in total, including 30 hospitals, 63 public health centers and 4 Women & Children's Health Centers, as well as 10,004 medical professionals, of whom 4,447 are doctors. The city provides 6,429 hospital beds. It also has established the Cooperative Health Care System in 481 villages by which 1.2 million rural people are covered for basic health care expenses.

The Psychiatric Clinic at the Third People's Hospital in Jian'an City

In 2005, the Psychiatric Clinic at the Third People's Hospital was the only clinic that provides diagnosis, treatment and hospital beds for the mentally ill in Jian'an City. My cousin, who was working at another local hospital, introduced me to the director of this clinic, Dr. Du. They used to attend medical school together. Their friendship from old days helped me get access to this clinic to do my research.

Compared to the First and Second People's Hospitals in Jian'an, the Third is quite small in its size and scale. The whole hospital only has one seven-floor building with a cheap looking outward appearance. Without the title plate hanging on the main entrance gate, the hospital could be easily mistaken for an inexpensive hotel. Walking into the lobby of the building, I found the arrangement to be almost the same as I can see at most hospitals in China. On my right was an information desk behind which there were many photos of people's faces lining the wall. Those faces are directors of all the clinics in this hospital. Pass the information desk and make a left, and you will see a corridor with many clinic rooms on both sides, of which three are occupied by the Psychiatric Clinic: two for interviewing outpatients, the third one for lab tests.

The Psychiatric Clinic of the Third People's Hospital was established in 1992. It had 5 doctors, 7 nurses and 60 hospital beds at the time when I was doing my field research there. Five doctors each work in the outpatient service, and shift each half-year. Outpatient service is open from 8 am to 5 pm, Monday to Friday.

Dr. Du is a tall young man, wearing a pair of golden-rimmed eyeglasses. He and his fellows started to work at this clinic in 1995. Before that, some people from other cities had been running it. As for those predecessors, Dr. Du told me, "Those guys are swindlers. They have no idea what mental illness is. They did nothing but cheat patients for money." Dr. Du told me that those "swindlers" signed a contract with the hospital to run this clinic, and each month they submitted part of their income. Before Dr. Du and his fellows told me this, I had never expected that this kind of commercial contract could have happened in a hospital. But it begins to make sense when considering the broader social context in which the radical transformation toward the market economy is swallowing up all of Chinese society. The medical system is no exception. Hospitals and other health care facilities have to struggle to make money like other institutions in order to survive the increasing competition in the market. For many hospitals, especially those small ones such as the Third People's Hospital in Jian'an, leasing the clinic might be a practical and easy decision to make. But to assess the results from marketizing the medical system is never going to be easy. In the context of martketizing the medical system, seeking health care turned into medicine shopping on the patients' part; while making money came to be a major concern of various medical institutions. The marketization of the medical system has placed people's health and the credibility of the medical system at great risk for which no one is going to take the ultimate responsibility. In today's China, worsening health inequality, increasing tension between doctors and patients, and spreading public health issues are widely articulated; more and more lawsuits concerning medical issues are occurring; the Chinese daily perceptions of the medical system barely appears positive. It is not known yet what kind of role this practice of leasing the clinic has played during a period when health inequality and doctor–patient relationship worsened and the credibility of the medical system has come to be questioned; but it is reasonable to believe that this practice made its significant contribution to some extent.

After Dr. Du and I got to know each other, Dr. Du said, "I happened to know your advisor. A few years ago I attended one of his lectures held in Beijing. His point sounds interesting to me. He seems to argue that social regime is the major cause of mental illness." The lecture Dr. Du mentioned was an academic workshop, which, as a form of short-term professional trainings offered within the medical system, is often held in big cities. It has been playing a major role in regulating local medical practices and updating the knowledge of those medical professionals working in small towns who barely have access to the latest information and technology. In China, there are big disparities between urban areas and rural areas, big cities and small towns, which make a great difference with respect to medical services, including medical equipment and medical staff's professional capability, available in different local places. The medical service available in small towns like Jian'an is not even close to what is offered in big cities such as Beijing and Shanghai. The academic workshops mentioned above have been contributing to the efforts of reducing these disparities, at least in terms of medical information and professional knowledge. However, it is not known how successful knowledge transfer is, so I was not sure how up-to-date and professionally competent Dr. Du and his colleagues were.

The Outpatient Clinic: Psychiatric or Psychological?

I noticed that the psychiatric clinic of the Third People's Hospital has two interview rooms with different doorplates hanging above the doors: one is "jingshen ke" (psychiatric clinic), and another is "xinli ke" (psychological clinic). Dr. Zhang was working in the outpatient service that day. He told me, "Even today many people do not understand what mental illness is and are afraid to go to a psychiatric clinic even when they have mental illness. Sometimes they refused to come in when they saw the doorplate, but they feel much better about the name psychological clinic. Thus, we have to arrange two interview rooms for outpatients; generally we are receiving outpatients in the psychological clinic room." Then Dr. Zhang proceeded to tell me a real story regarding this arrangement of the two interview rooms. A patient came to consult about his mental problem, and Dr. Zhang directed him into the room with the doorplate of jingshen ke. The patient suddenly noticed the doorplate when he was entering the room. He immediately jumped out of the doorway and complained, "This is jingshen ke, isn't it? I'm not psychotic. Do you think I'm crazy? You must be wrong. This is ridiculous. I am not going in there. No way!"

The arrangement of two interview rooms with different doorplates and those stories that have happened behind that arrangement reveal to us the Chinese lay view of mental illness and its powerful effect in Chinese local life worlds. People's fear of the term mental illness implies the strong stigma related to this illness. In China, lay people view mental illness (jingshen bing) as a chronic, serious and incurable disease, while psychological illness (xinli bing) is thought as an acute, minor and curable mental problem. Besides these two lay terms describing mental health problems, shenjingbing, literally translated as neurosis but carrying the same meaning as "nuts" does in English, is another term widely used in Chinese daily life. In contrast to its literal meaning, the term shenjingbing conveys the idea of psychosis and insanity. It refers to a person with psychotic behavior no matter the source. With a strongly derogatory meaning, this term has been used to label anyone whose behavior is not accepted as normal or reasonable, or is extremely annoying. Therefore, shenjingbing, as a label, is basically applied to two groups: people who have real mental illness, and those who act like the mentally ill but do not have an illness.

Chinese lay views of mental health problem can be traced back to the theoretical framework of traditional Chinese medicine and its explanation of mental illness. Traditional Chinese medicine has a holistic view of humans, the environment and the cosmos; none can be separated from each other. Instead, the external and the inside, mind and body interact with each other and constitute circulation with no end. Smooth circulation leads to the balance or harmony of Yin/Yang and Five Elements, which is the fundamental idea of health in traditional Chinese medicine. When circulation becomes excessive or insufficient, the micro and macro interaction cannot work smoothly or has shut down, the balance or harmony of the whole is broken, and then people get sick. In terms of the etiology of traditional Chinese medicine, imbalance and stagnation are the original causes of illness.

In traditional Chinese medical literatures, dian (similar to depression) and kuang (similar to craziness) were named as two types of mental disorders. The conceptions of dian and kuang came from *Lingshu-dian kuang*. Dian features excessive yin while kuang features excessive yang (*Nanjing*, Han Dynasty). According to *Danxixinfa-dian kuang* (Xiaojun zhengheng, Yuan Dynasty), both dian and kuang are caused by stagnation of phlegm within chest, which is the somatization of the stagnation of emotions. To quote *Zhengzhiyaojue* (Dai Yuanli, volume 9) of Ming Dynasty, "Dian and kuang are both caused by the stagnation of emotions". Meanwhile, vomiting was believed to be the treatment. However, traditional Chinese medicine has never tried to sharpen the distinction between dian and kuang, instead it insists that neither dian nor kuang has exclusive symptoms, rather these two diseases can mutually transform into each other during the disease course. Traditional Chinese medicine also suggests that mental disorders have a close relationship to individual's congenital character and physical constitution, which explains the existence of family illness history of dian and kuang, and also provides an explanation to why some people develop dian or kuang while others do not in the face of similar emotional stagnation.

Examining today's lay views of mental disorder in China, we can still single out the influence and remains of traditional Chinese medical theories, such as the stagnation theory and the emphasis on the possible relationship of mental illness to individual's congenital character and physical constitution. In general, people believe that mental disorder is caused by emotional stagnation stimulated by some critical events or situations. In this view, if people's physical or psychological constitution is too weak to bear strong emotional stimulations, they cannot pass through the emotional stagnation, and then their mental structures will shut down and they cannot function as normal persons. When it comes to some people trapped in emotional stagnation, Chinese say that he/she just cannot think through (xiang bu tong). In Chinese daily sayings, emotional stagnations are always called heart knot (xin jie). If one cannot untie a heart knot successfully, one cannot think through it, there is no chance that he/she can resolve emotional stagnation. Moreover, people assume that a normal person should be able to untie a heart knot and eliminate emotional stagnation sooner or later. If the person failed to do so, it means that the person must have had some physical or psychological weaknesses or defects that make the person not function as a normal person. Here we can see that there is a tendency to refuse to acknowledge mental disorder as a real disease in Chinese culture. People rather tend to regard mental disorder as a temporary minor physical or psychological problem that a normal person should be able to overcome and resolve by him/herself. If it becomes an irresolvable chronic problem, there must be something wrong with the person who has this problem. Hence the person him/herself should be questioned and blamed for his/her problem.

The Inpatient Department

The Inpatient Department for the mentally ill at the Third People's Hospital took up the entire seventh floor of the hospital building. It had an iron door with a keeper on watch. Walking up to the seventh floor, talking to the keeper through a video intercom, I was allowed to get into the ward area. On my right there was an observation room, which was also the doctor's office and nurse's station. On my left there was an open space in which a table-tennis table was set up. The observation room had a big window facing the open space. At the other end of the open space there were about 10 wardrooms lined on both sides by a long corridor. Each ward had six beds and six closets. Under each bed a plastic washbowl was placed on the ground. Everything was white except for the different colors of those washbowls.

More than 40 patients were hospitalized at the time when I was doing my field research there. The moment I walked into the ward area, several nurses were distributing medicine in the open space, and dozens of patients were waiting in a line besides the table-tennis table. Some patients were walking around without any purpose; others were sitting on the ground with their backs against the wall while staring at nothing. Nurses put medicine in a small plastic bottle and handed it to each patient, watched the patient take the medicine, then asked the patient to open the mouth to check if he/she had taken the medicine. Then the next patient in line came up to undergo the same medicine-taking process.

Stigma Among the Stigmatized — She's Nuts! We Are Not

A patient approached me when I was wandering around in the ward area. He appeared very young, in grey shirt, yellow pants and worn sandals. We then started to converse outside one of the wardrooms. He expressed great interest in me and was curious about where I came from and what I was doing in there. He kept looking down to floor and never made eye contact while speaking with me. He also kept bending his body back and forth rhythmically. I soon noticed that he always tried to move the left side of his body toward me even if I had to alter my position in order to talk to him face to face. I invited him into a wardroom so that we could seat ourselves on a bed and talk at ease. He sat down with me for only a few seconds before standing up again. "I have to stand up", he said. We continued our conversation standing for the rest of the time. This young man, whose name is Wen, told me that he once was a high school student and was very interested in computers. As Wen said, he was hospitalized because that he simply could not concentrate his mind on anything. To quote his words, "I have a neurosis, but I am trying to get away from it. Once I recover, I would like to be a computer-technician."

When we were talking, another patient walked in. Wen introduced me to this new comer, Luo, who was of Wen's age. Luo stood against me and kept rubbing his hands, revealing nervousness. I tried to ease his mind by patting his shoulder and welcoming him to join us. Luo started to talk, "you don't have to talk to others, they are all psychotic. We two just have neurosis, we are not insane." Wen nodded and aligned himself with Luo, "they are all crazy". While we were chatting, another patient, a girl, stepped in and grasped my backpack all of a sudden. I said hello to her, but she kept holding my backpack without verbal response. Wen came and helped me pull her hands off while Luo pushed her on her shoulders. They teased the girl, saying to me, "she is nuts. Do not talk to her. She knows nothing." They fought over my backpack for a while, and then the girl gave up and left. Wen and Luo said, "she is a real shenjingbing." It did not take more than a few minutes before Luo manifested no more interest in the conversation. Wen, who apparently noticed it, then said to me, "You have to pat him again, otherwise, he is never going to leave. That is what his neurosis is about. If one touched him, the same one has to do that again to dismiss him. Or he will just remain that way forever." So I had to follow Wen's instruction to let Luo go. No surprise, Luo walked away happy.

At the time when Dr. Yang was responsible for treating them, I once asked about Wen and Luo and was informed that both of them were diagnosed with schizophrenia. I further asked him how patients themselves viewed their own illnesses. Dr. Yang smiled and replied, "A lot of people do not understand what mental illness is. Few admit that they have it; rather, they always describe fellow patients to be actually mentally ill. And patients' families also feel about mental illness in the same way." Apparently, Dr. Yang was not interested at all in how patients themselves feel about their own diseases. Instead he continued to prove his argument of patients' families being ignorant about mental illness by telling me a story that once occurred in his clinic. A couple brought in their son for diagnosis, the doctor on duty concluded that the boy was in a serious condition and had to be hospitalized immediately. The parents then became nervous and, despite their eventual compliance with the doctor's suggestion, requested to first take a look at the ward. They wanted to make sure the ward was good for their son to stay. With the permission from the doctor, the parents went upstairs to check out the ward. After a few minutes they came back angry and shouted at the doctor, "Are you out of your mind? Those people are shenjingbing. How can you put our son there with those madmen? Our son is not shenjingbing. He just has a little xinli bing. I will never let my son stay there. You are totally messed up." They then left with their son, and never came back.

The story told by Dr. Yang once again confirmed that Chinese tend to reject and deny the concept of mental illness when it applies to themselves and others who are close to them. The issue that interested me, however, is how patients understand their own problems and treat each other. Wen and Luo's contrasts with other patients makes me believe that besides medical professionals, patients themselves also classify diseases and label each other. Moreover, patients' classifying and labeling behavior is about the embodiment of stigma associated with mental illness. It shows that the stigmatized is not, in fact, monolithic; rather, it is also divided between the stigmatizers and the stigmatized, meaning that stigma even exists within the stigmatized group, which verifies the existence of the stigmatization of the stigmatized. To this fact the theory of internalization of stigma might be a possible explanation. But according to the conclusion derived from research on internalization of stigma to date, it is supposed to lead to self-stigmatization rather than to stigmatize other stigmatized. It is my concern to explore this issue later.

Stigma Within a Local Work Unit — They Avoid, Tease and Make Fun of Me

Jianguo was the first patient I formally interviewed at the Psychiatric Clinic of the Third People's Hospital in Jian'an. By that time, he had been hospitalized for three months. Born in a rural family in western Hubei, Jianguo is the second eldest of four children in his family. He graduated from Wuhan Metallurgy College in 1990, which really surprised me because he looked like a farmer who had never left his village rather than someone who had attended college. He was 36 years old but looked much older because of his gray hair. We were sitting in a wardroom. He was very shy and did not talk much.

In 1994 when he was working in Jian'an, Jianguo was hospitalized for the first time. Regarding the onset of his illness, Jianguo told me an interesting story. "That day I was playing outside, all of a sudden the Earth was shaking somehow. I immediately had a strong feeling that the Earth is going to leave the solar system at that moment." Jianguo was a little embarrassed by his own story but finally started to talk at ease.

"I was not worried about that", he continued, "Because I knew there were other stars even if we left the solar system. But I just cannot stop thinking about it. That really bothered me." The other thing haunting Jianguo, as he said, was disaster brought by the explosion of Atomic and Hydrogen bombs that come from nowhere. He could not help thinking about these things, not until he fell asleep because of exhaustion resulting from thinking. Finally Jianguo became psychotic while he was working. Jianguo's co-workers took him to this hospital; later on he was diagnosed with schizophrenia and then hospitalized. After several months, Jianguo seemed to have recovered from his illness. He left the hospital and went back to work. But things soon became worse. Jianguo has been hospitalized intermittently since then.

After talking for a while, I asked Jianguo once again what he thinks caused his illness. This time he attributed his illness to interference and disturbance from outside. "They (Jianguo's work fellows) always pay too much attention to me. They kept watching me and talking about me," Jianguo said. He felt his co-workers were stalking and peeking in on him everywhere, and he could not stop thinking that his co-workers were talking about him behind his back and trying to hurt him.

After college, Jianguo was assigned to work for a well-known construction company in Shanghai. After several months, he was reassigned to a branch company in Wuhan. He could not keep the job longer than a month until he was reassigned once again to a local construction company in Jian'an city. Jianguo attributed his dramatically downward social mobility from Shanghai to Wuhan and then on to Jian'an (from the most modern city of China to the capital of Hubei province, and then on to a small town) as his problematic personality. As he said, he always has difficulty in handling interpersonal relationships and social networks, which he regards as too complicated for him. To quote his words, "I am not a people person. I would rather read a book or think about something at home alone than go out with my friends or co-workers." When he was talking, he was staring at something on the ground, seeming to speak to himself with a shy smile on his face. He said that he always had a problem getting along with his co-workers or developing good relations with the leaders of his work unit. "I just don't know what to do and how to do it when it comes to these things."

"My work mates used to tease and make fun of me, which drove me crazy." Jianguo continued, "I always take everything too seriously. When I was with my co-workers, I could not tell when they were joking or telling the truth. I guess they all think I'm dumb and stupid. They often make fun of me, and fool around like I am a funny idiot. If you are introversive and not good at developing relations, they disdain and ignore you. They never treat you as a person with social face." When he was telling me this, Jianguo seemed not angry at the way his co-workers had been treating him; rather, he always had that shy smile on his face while playing with the lower hem corner of his shirt.

"Things became even worse after I was hospitalized because of my mental illness." Jianguo went on to tell me a story about how he was fooled by his co-workers. One day when he was working, one of his co-workers stopped by and said to him, "hey, boss wants to talk to you, he is waiting for you at his office. Hurry up." Then Jianguo ran into his boss's office and found out his boss was in the middle of a conference. His boss seemed to have no idea why he was there. Jianguo was getting confused but still told his boss what he had heard from his co-worker, and then his boss became angry and shouted at him, "who said I want to talk to you? Nonsense, get out! I don't have time for this!" Jianguo was completely lost and could not figure out what was going on, and then he went back and told the same co-worker what just happened. The guy burst into laughter and said, "I cannot believe you are such a dumb ass. There is no such talk at all. Don't you get it? How could the boss want to talk to you? Talk to you about what? You are nuts! Don't you know that?" Eventually, Jianguo found out that his co-worker lied to him and had played with him.

Jianguo's co-workers repeated the same trick on him again and again and again. Sometimes they made a little change to the plot. For example, they once told Jianguo that some girl, also one of his co-workers, always likes him but is too shy to say it to his face; when Jianguo's face turned red, they went on to say that the girl would like to meet him at some place sometime, and then they even pretended to encourage or force Jianguo to go to the date that does not exist. When Jianguo arrived at the place on time, of course, he found nobody.

Besides this trick, Jianguo's work mates have other ways to make fun of Jianguo. In his presence, they often mention the explosion of atomic or hydrogen bomb since they know that this is going to scare him. They would suddenly shout at Jianguo, "hey, a bomb is going to blow right away, is it atomic or hydrogen?" They deliberately do so for fun: when Jianguo became scared and started to talk nonsense, they burst into laughter. They love to repeat this any time they want. Some of Jianguo's work fellows criticize others for doing this to him, but they never try to stop them, rather they also enjoy watching the show when it gets to its climax. "When they do so, I feel extremely scared. My heart starts to beat very fast and I begin to sweat. And what I can hear is only a voice talking within my head, 'run! run! run! It is going to explode,' which makes me dizzy and nauseous, I can hardly breathe, and then I started to run around to find place to hide."

After his hospitalization due to mental illness, all of his co-workers began to avoid him; none would like to work with him on the same project; they did not even want to sit next to him when they were eating at the company's dining room. One thing that has never changed is that they continue to tease and make fun of him. In his work unit, nobody treated Jianguo as a person with dignity; besides that, his co-workers also used him as a monster to scare somebody else because some work fellows, especially those girls known for being timid, are afraid to get close to him. Sometimes, Jianguo's co-workers pushed him around to get in the way of those girls, who then became scared, started to scream and run away. They also used Jianguo to make fun of some girls by saying, "hey, I heard that you are seeing Jianguo. Somebody saw you being with him last weekend," or like, "hey, Jianguo told me that he likes you and wants to date you."

Jianguo has been living in isolation. He has never been in a relationship or married. "Before I had this illness, I was too shy, nobody would like to be with me. After that, my illness scares everyone away when they hear about it. There is no chance that a mentally ill could find someone to get married. This is the reality. You have to take it no matter what you want. If you have mental illness, you are completely stranded. There is no job, no marriage, no future, and no hope at all. I feel lucky that I still keep my job and my company covers my medical expense because my company is owned by the state and they cannot fire people. Otherwise I must have already lost my job. That is for sure. You see lots of things going on everyday in the world, but you have nothing to do with them. You have nothing to do with anything."

Jianguo has been living alone in Jian'an since he came to work there in 1991. His hometown is about four hundred kilometers away. The rest of his family members including his parents, brothers and sisters are all living in the same village where they were born and still farming. Jianguo's family came to see him several times when he was previously hospitalized. "They do care about me, but there is nothing they can do to help me get out of this. There is no way out."

"Have they come to see you recently?" I asked.

"Not yet. I do not even know if they got the information that I am hospitalized again. My company used to send a message to my family if I am hospitalized. I am not sure if they did that this time. My family is far away from here. They are all farmers and do not make much money. It would cost them more money than what they can make to come to see me. Thus, it is not even easy for them to afford visiting me even once." Jianguo said, with a permanent shy smile on his face.

In Jianguo's case, I observe that, his illness, in his work mate's view, is not just a psychological or mental disease in medical sense; instead it became a problem with his whole person, which came to be an inherent part of his life experience. To some extent, Jianguo's illness experience became all of his life experience.

Before he was diagnosed with schizophrenia and hospitalized, Jianguo had already been stigmatized because his difficulty in dealing with interpersonal relationship and developing good social network. His life experience provides a typical example of members of marginal groups living in today's China. In the face of radical social competition, his rural family background could not provide any substantial support for him, while his introversion further put him into a disadvantageous position. His illness experience is an embodiment of his whole social experience: he has been isolated, suppressed and haunted by his illness as well as by the social context in which he has been living. Jianguo blames others (co-workers) for causing his illness and blame himself (his personality) for his own unsuccessful work experience. His downward social movement is the fate of workers of marginal groups in the face of rapid social transformation: a kind of social Darwinism — selection through severe social competition. In this situation, there is no chance that marginal groups could speak out about or resist the structural violence of society. What they can do is to blame themselves and to attribute their failure to their own weaknesses and defects. They regard their failures as an unavoidable and inescapable fate resulting from their poor family background and the consequent inability to make good social relations and develop valuable social networks.

Social face, social relations and networks are major concepts when it comes to study Chinese society. So far, many researchers working in this field contend that these concepts have been playing significant roles in Chinese local life world and they are keys to understand Chinese daily behavior, local communities and the whole society. Despite the fact that the alleged assumption that these concepts are exclusive to Chinese society is itself questionable, however, most of researchers to date have been focusing on the management of social face, social relations and networks, especially on how Chinese successfully make social face and manage good social relations and networks in their local life world. Notably, stigma presents us a new angle to look into these issues, that is, what it is like when people fail to make social face or manage social relations and networks.

In Chinese cultural context, social face, similar to the idea of yang sheng (fostering health rather than maintaining health) in traditional Chinese medicine, is not a given or static social status but something varying according to one's daily practices of cultural norms. By different practices, one either makes or loses social face, which depends on one's understanding of cultural norms and application of particular practices in specific situations. The daily practices of cultural norms consist mainly of making social relations, and establishing and further developing social networks. Social face is based on social relations and social networks: powerful social relations and social networks make strong social face; lack of social relations and social networks makes no social face, which deprives a person of the right to live respectfully and to be treated as a normal person. In general, people do not disface a person what has social face because the latter has social resources to fight back and disface the former. Social face is what makes a human being a person; lack of social face reduces a person into non-person.

In Jianguo's case, he has difficulty in getting along with his work fellows and developing good relations with the leaders of his work unit. He lives as a person without social relations and outside any social network; moreover, he has further been denied his opportunity to change this situation because of his mental illness. Jianguo's experience within his work unit makes it very clear that he is avoided, disdained, and teased by his work fellows because of his inability to develop social relations and his lack of social networks and his mental illness only make his situation even worse. When Jianguo failed to make social relations and establish social networks, he lost the ability to make social face and became a non-person; meanwhile, his co-workers perceive him as a non-person without social face, which allowed them impunity. They do not feel guilty because they disdain, tease, stigmatize and discriminate against him. In the Chinese context, for the stigmatized, stigma results from lack of social face caused by absence of social relations and a shutdown of social networks; for the stigmatizers, people stigmatize someone because they perceive he or she is a non-person who does not deserve to be treated as a normal person with social face and dignity.

Stigma Within a Village — They Do Not Invite Me to Family Events Anymore

One morning, while I was talking to Dr. Zhang at his outpatient clinic, a middle-aged man, Dong, came in to pick up medicine for his wife who has depression. I explained my research to Dong and asked if I could visit his family. Dong was hesitant but eventually agreed. Thirty minutes later

I was sitting on the backseat of his small motorbike traveling toward his home, which is in a village about twenty kilometers from downtown. On the way to his home, I asked Dong about his wife's condition. It turned out that his wife of 44 years old had been suffering depression since 1993.

"What do you think depression is? How do you feel about it?"

"I am not a doctor, I don't really know about it. But in my perspective, my wife has been worrying about too many things. Her brain is too developed, while the developed things are likely to have problems. That's the why she got sick. My point is, more developed the society is, more things people need to think about, and more troubles they are going to have." He was driving, turning his face to me and asking, "Do you agree with me? "

Then he added, "Those idiots will never have this kind of illness because they never think. What do you say? Am I correct?"

. . .

The motorbike's engine was so noisy that we had to shout at each other to continue our conversation on local knowledge about the etiology of depression.

Thirty minutes later, we left the national road and turned on to a rugged alley in the field. We arrived at his home after another thirty minutes. There was a level open space in front of his house. A fishpond was on the left and a pigsty on the right. Dong's wife was not in at the time we arrived. He said, "She is not comfortable with staying at home alone. If she saw nobody else at home, she would go out and walk around without any purpose. She is afraid of being at home alone."

While waiting for his wife, Dong showed me around his house. They have a small size field for farming rice. In addition, he has been running a fishpond, a pigsty and a fruit garden for years in order to make extra money for family financial support. In 2002, they built a pigsty and raised more than twenty pigs for sale. The following year they rebuilt the pigsty and raised more than forty pigs. Dong said, "I have to run some sidelines like these to make extra money. If we just farm, we could never keep up with increased family expenses including medical fees and children's school tuition." In the 1970s, sideline, absolutely prohibited in rural areas because of communistic ideology, was regarded as "the tail of capitalism" that must be cut off with all private-running business. Over the subsequent

"Reform and Open" period starting since the late 1970s, "developing sideline in rural areas" was announced by the central government as a nationwide policy that aimed to lift rural families out of poverty, called fa jia zhi fu (to increase the family fortunes and become rich). Sideline became a major way by which some rural families earn extra money to build themselves new houses and buy modern furniture and electronic equipment, from wristwatch, bicycle and sewing machine in the 1970s to TV set, washing machine, refrigerator, and motorcycle in the 1980s. Those families who were good at running sidelines became "wan yuan hu", (households with yearly income of ten thousand yuan) who were praised as the leaders of the "becoming rich" campaign launched by government at all rural levels. After the 1990s, sideline business came to be a must-have financial support for rural families to maintain basic daily living. "The society and the policies made by the government are changing too fast; you will never keep up with the pace of change," Dong commented.

Dong and his wife have two children, one son and one daughter. A few years ago, the son dropped out of high school and went to da gong (doing part-time work submitted to short-term and flexible contract) in Jian'an to make money. "It is useless to attend school these days. You spend lots of money in school, but you could still hardly find a job after you finished your schooling. For a family like us, you'd better get out of school to make money as soon as you can. Otherwise it would be a huge waste of money. I told my children so, but my daughter just does not listen to me." Dong sighed. His daughter was still attending high school; she was living in school's dorm and only came home on weekends. "Sometimes my daughter does not come home on weekends. Even if she came back, she would like to stick to her friends rather than stay at home and help us do some housework, in part because she is ashamed of her mother's illness. You should know what is going to happen when you have this kind of illness. Those silly people tease and disdain you when you have a mentally ill family member. Sometimes it makes your life really hard, you simply cannot ignore it. You have to live with it."

Walking into the living room, their daughter's bedroom was on the left and the son's bedroom on the right. The parents place their bedroom outside next to the pigsty in the big yard because at nights they have to watch the pigs they are raising. "Stealing pigs occurs a lot in villages; we have to watch out day and night. We are really counting on those pigs to make some money."

When we were sitting and talking in the living room, Dong's wife, Guiying, came home. At her first sight of her husband, she started to complain, "Where have you been? I came back from the field and did not see you. I was so scared and wondering where you were going. I just cannot stay at home alone, so I went out." She is a typical middle-aged rural Chinese woman, short, thin and swarthy, revealing her long-term of hard work in the field. After she sat down, Guiying started to bring out her medicine bottles one by one and kept asking me about her medicine, never heeding my introduction of the research project. Unfortunately, I could not tell her more than what I read from the instruction attached to her medicine bottles, explaining that I was not a medical doctor.

Before she married to Dong, Guiying had been working as a tailor in the county town for several years. By doing so she saved some money for herself. In 1984, after Dong and Guiying married, Guiying quit the tailor's job and stayed at home, devoting most of her time to farming and housework. The following year they built a new house for themselves, which made this family stand out from the rest of the families in the village. They were admired and envied by their neighbors. "Truly, that was a great time!" said Guiying, thinking back to those days. All those good memories seemed to have come back to her at that moment. "But good days are always short. You never know what is ahead of you." Guiying soon came back to reality with a long sigh.

In 1993, one night, Dong's father, a doorman working in Jian'an city, died in an accident. It happened all of a sudden, Dong and all of the family's relatives except for Guiying and her two children rushed to Jian'an to take care of the body and prepare funeral arrangements. Guiying, as she said, had to stay at home to look after her two children who were very young at the time. That night Guiying began acting crazy.

"I was not there when she went crazy; none of our relatives was at home. Nobody knew what happened to her. Later I heard from villagers that she kept talking, jumping, singing in nonsense, charging in and out of the house, and running around in the fields. Some villagers had to chase her around the village to get her. When they finally did, four young men took her home and bound her to the bed. She was terribly crazy and some neighbors had to watch her for the whole night. At the time we did not have home phone or cell phone. There was no way that our neighbors could have informed me about this that night. The following day, they sent someone to Jian'an to tell me about this." Dong added, "it almost drove me crazy too. You know, my father just died and my wife went crazy at the same time. Misfortune never singly comes."

Guiying was hospitalized for almost a month. After that, her illness recurred several times. Whenever something bad happened to this family, her illness would recur.

"I could not go to sleep at nights, and I felt my head is going to explode. Sometimes I felt dizzy, and I always feel someone is laughing at me. My head is bloated and in pain." Guiying was talking with her hands around her head, and then she posed her right hand as a knife to chop her head, saying, "Sometimes it is so painful that I wish I could cut off my own head, and then I won't feel the pain."

After she got sick, Guiying came to be afraid of staying at home alone. If she had not seen her husband for a while, she would have had a feeling of "guo bu de" (having something stuck in one's heart and feeling one cannot pass through that moment). Then she had to leave home and went to her relatives's place to stay with them. Owing to her illness, she has to reduce her workload. Once her illness recurred, she had to stop working for two months. "I used to work on everything and had never felt tired; but now I am likely to get tired, which makes me feel I am useless to this family. There is a lot of housework needed to be done, but I just cannot help."

Guiying's most recent illness relapse was caused by her son's lawsuit. After he dropped out of high school, the boy went to work as a handicraftsman in Jian'an city. Unfortunately, he happened to be hired by a cold-hearted boss. Having worked for a month, the boy could not get the money he was promised because his boss refused to pay him for no reason. The young boy became angry and planned revenge on his boss. He stole his boss's cell phone and wanted to sell it for money to make up the payment he thought he deserve to get from his boss. When he was trying to sell the cell phone on the street, he got caught and was arrested by the police. The judge said the boy could be put on probation for a fine of 3,000 yuan. Guiying went mad again when she heard this news.

Guiying said she always feels scared even if nothing has happened. She was too scared to go to sleep at night. "I did not do anything, but I'm fearful all the time," she said. She seemed to have no clue how to control her fear. But her husband cut in and said, "You just like to think too much! As I told you before, if you could put those nonsense aside and stop thinking, you would feel better and get on with your life. Your illness could disappear immediately!" Guiying raised her voice in anger and replied, "I know I should have controlled my mind not to think too much, but I just cannot stop thinking. If I know how to stop it, I won't complain any more. You just don't understand. You have no idea about how I feel because you are not me!" Guiying's husband's local knowledge of mental illness can be rephrased as the following: suffering comes from the development of society that causes excessive mental activities, in his words, too much thinking. Rethinking suffering reproduces more suffering. However, suffering, in Guiying's perspective, results from the painful sediment ingrained in her body, memory, and every corner of her daily life over those past years.

There is little question that all of these factors, including family financial problem, loss of family members, and her son's lawsuit, together contributed to Guiying's endless fear. She has been living in fear, which results from the feeling of being unsafe and insecure caused by a series of unfortunate family events. Each relapse of her illness marks each misfortune that has happened to her family. Guiying's mental illness poses not only a burden onto her family, including increased medical fees and loss of manpower in housework, farming, and family sidelines, but also a challenge to the whole family about how to face up to it and outcome, and also how to get on with their lives with the stigma related to her mental illness in the village.

Without a word to his wife about her complaints, Dong turned away to work on something else; Guiying went on to complain how some of the villagers made fun of her after they uncovered her mental illness. Guiying's psychotic behavior that night also made her mental illness known by everyone in the village. There was no chance that the family could have hid her mental illness from the rest of the villagers. Sometimes when she runs into others in village, "they stop and stare at me, saying that someone in my family is in trouble since they know I am likely to go crazy if I hear of any bad news concerning my family. They just like to watch how scared I become and then laugh at me," said Guiying. Her husband added, "Those people are senseless and mean. They just love to scare her for fun. You know, rural people are rude; they don't have any sense of being nice to each other. For example, they would say to her: hey, your father-in-law just died or your husband/son/daughter got into trouble." Guiying had been overwhelmed by a series of family misfortunes and could not take any more bad news; while those villagers like to simulate the overwhelming situation, force her to relive that painful experience, and then watch how she suffers from that situation.

I asked about their relations to relatives. "They are still nice to me. Sometimes I went to their places and stay with them for a while. They used to come in a lot to chat with me if they had time; but after I got sick, they seldom come to see me except for on festival days. I understand that. Anyway, I, after all, have this illness, which is not something good," Guiying replied with a bitter smile.

"Then what about your family's relation with your neighbors and other villagers? Has it ever changed since you had this illness?"

"That is a different story. I can feel that they intend to avoid me. I did not feel that way right after I got sick, but later on I found out that they regard me as different. The way they look at and talk to me both make me feel that I am different in their eyes. Sometimes when I saw they were chatting together, I feel like joining them, but once I was there, standing or sitting next to them, they would not talk in the same way as they did without me. They would keep changing topics and also talked less. During the talk, I can feel that they were peeking in on me from time to time. I can immediately feel the tension comes out suddenly, which also makes me nervous and do not know what to say. I tried several times; it has never worked. After that I gave up and now I am getting used to stay by myself."

"After you got sick, have they ever invited you to any family event, such as wedding or funeral, as they did before?"

"No, they do not do that anymore. We used to help each other on these things. When you have a wedding or funeral at your family, you just let me know and I will go over to help everything, such as receiving guests, cooking meals, and washing utensils. It is very common in the village.

People feel they are honored when they are invited to help on the scene, even that work could be exhaustive; if you were not invited, it would be a shame on you. It means that the host family of the events looks down on you and does not care about your social face because they feel comfortable to disface you by not inviting you; or they think you are improper for the events and your presence would disface themselves. That is how these things work in the village. They did invite me before I got sick; but after that, they intend to ignore or avoid me. They do not inform me about these events any more. Well, I know it is because of my mental illness, but you can say nothing about it. There is no issue of social face at all when you become mentally ill. Nobody care how you feel. You have no rights to argue or complain about the way you are being treated. You have little choice but to accept it."

Guiying's eyes teared, she went on, "But there are some people who are good at zuo ren (always be a nice person, good at handling all kinds of social relations and never disface anyone). They tell me about the events and invite me to help because they are trying to be nice and do not want to disface me by not telling or ignoring me. But they, in fact, already knew that I am not going to be there. It is a common sense, how couldn't I know that? I am ok with that. If they are nice to me and do not want to disface me, how can I go there to disface them in public? So I just find an excuse and tell them I cannot make it."

The internalization of stigma might be a convenient explanation of Guiying's turning down the invitation, namely, she does not want to attend the events because of shame; but there is more in this situation that needs to be noted and analyzed. To understand whether or not to attend a ceremony event in the Chinese context, one has to take guanxi and renqing into account. According to Yan (1996), guanxi refers to social relationships and social networks and renqing (human feelings) is a system of ethics based on commonsense knowledge of sharing and face. Yan further defines sharing as the moral basis of renqing (1996:128) and face as the moral constraint in social interaction (1996:133). For sharing, "one side was obligated to offer and the other had a claim or right to receive," refusing to share "usually is considered selfish and unsocial" (1996:132). Hence, a family is obligated to host a ceremony to share their happiness (like in a wedding) or sadness (like in a funeral) with the others in the community. In his research of gift exchange in a Chinese village, Yan mentions "dead doors", which refers to those "who do not cultivate such [guanxi] networks" and therefore "are relegated to socially disadvantaged positions" (1996:103). Dead doors are persons who have "failed to establish a respectable place for himself or herself in the society, thus showing a lack of knowledge of what it means to be a human being" (1996:103). Yan further points out that "the disadvantages of failing in social exchange and network building are not limited to verbal expression — there are also social sanctions. Most commonly, those who cannot fulfill the obligations of gift giving and other forms of social exchange are isolated by the majority in the village, and during personal crises this isolation becomes a serious social sanction" (1996:104). In order to show how dead doors are rejected and isolated in the village, Yan cites two cases: a young couple disliked the village life style "because of their higher education" and the husband being working in a city and "deliberately avoided attending village ceremonies and gradually isolated themselves" (1996:104), thus no one came to visit the wife when she underwent a sterilization operation; in another cases, a man who "does not talk much and isolates himself from the villagers" (1996:104) could not raise enough money for his son's wedding and had to take out a loan from someone from another village. In the end, only a few people attended the wedding and the gift money the host family received was less than usual. Yan uses the two cases to demonstrate "the significance of guanxi networks in the public area" (1996:105).

Looking back at Guiying's case, I have to say that she was definitely in the similar situation of dead doors. She was no longer invited to attend those ceremonies in the village after she had mental illness, which means that she had no more social sanction; namely, she was not socially recognized or accepted anymore in the village. But Guiying's story is different from Yan's cases in several aspects. First, Guiying was not the host of those ceremonies but the one who should have been invited and who had to decide whether to attend the ceremonies hosted by other families; while in Yan's cases, it was villagers that refused to attend the ceremonies held by dead doors. Second, in Yan's cases, it seems that dead doors isolated themselves because of their inflexible and unsocial personality, and then they are isolated by the villagers; while in Guiying's case, she was socially recognized and accepted until she had mental illness. That is to say, she did not isolate herself from the villagers; rather, she was isolated by the villagers after she was found psychotic. Therefore, Guiying's case shows that there is another type of dead doors in addition to that described by Yan. In Yan's model, the term of dead doors "symbolizes both the incapability and inflexibility of the persons and thus at a deeper level their social death in the domain of social exchange and network construction" (1996:103). Apparently, Guiying's social death was not a result of her incapability or inflexibility in making guanxi; rather, it was because that she was considered a person who already lost her ability to make guanxi because of her psychosis. If dead doors in Yan's cases are considered persons who lack the common sense knowledge of what it means to be a human being, then Guiying, in the villagers' opinion, became one who was not able to be a human being anymore after she was found psychotic. This is the very reason that she was no longer invited by other villagers to those ceremonies.

Although there were some villagers who did invite Guiying, she still decides not to accept the invitation because she noticed her social identity and status in the village after she had psychosis. She claimed that she did not want to disface those who still regarded her as a normal person with social face and invited her. By refusing to accept the invitation, she tried to show others that she still knew how face and guanxi work in the local life world; namely, she wanted show that she still had the common sense of renqing, which is to save face for one other. "The ethics of renqing requires those of lower rank to help protect the social face of those of higher rank" (1996:137). In this sense, if Guiying accepted the invitation and attended the ceremony, she would be considered a person who was not aware of her own social identity and who had no sense about the difference in the social status between her and those who invited her. Therefore, her decision of not attending those ceremonies reveals her concern for other's situation and her caring about other's face. She was trying to act as a person who is obligated to save face for others. Guiying's story reveals a dilemma confronting Guiying: she was considered a non-person but still tried to act as a person who knows about the issues of face and guanxi. The way Guiying managed her stigmatizing situation suggests that it was the stigma related to her mental illness that turned her into a non-person and forced her to isolate herself from the other villagers.

Yan also describes imbalance in gift exchange in China before 1949, which usually happens between tenants and landlords. "The Landlords might send a representative and offer a gift, but he did not come unless a special relationship had developed between the two parties" (1996:152). The difference in face, namely, "landlord's face was bigger than that of tenants", explains the absence of the landlord at the ceremonies (1996:152). In Guiying's case, her absence at the ceremonies apparently was not because she had bigger face than others because of her HIV/AIDS status. Yan further introduces the gift exchange in China after 1949 in a hierarchical model, in which subordinates play the role of giver and the gift flows upward and unilaterally while superiors are always receivers who have no obligation to return the gift. As Yan notes, in most cases, ordinary villagers would not send invitations to their superiors, "by so doing, they helped their superiors avoid the obligation of returning gifts" (1996:153). In Guiying's case, villagers did not send her invitation apparently not because she was their superiors. Yan points out that when people with higher social status host ceremonies, they do not care who come to attend the ceremony; rather, they only want to know "who has not attended the ritual" (1996:164), and then they have many ways to "express their anger toward those who fail to fulfill the obligation to give gifts" and punish them (1996:164). Guiying was not in this situation either. Nobody cared about whether she attended the ceremonies; in fact, they did not want her to be there and they wound not mind either if she did not show up with a gift. No one would bother to punish her for her absence. In this sense, in the villagers' opinion, Guiying even was not comparable to a person who was at the low level of social status system; rather, her situation was worse than that. She was excluded from the gift exchange networks, which means that she was not considered a person anymore.

Late that afternoon, I decided to finish the interview and leave Guiying's family. Dong found out that one of his neighbors, Zhao, a truck driver running his own business, could give me a ride back to downtown, but I had to wait for Zhao to finish loading his truck. Several villagers were chatting nearby, and I went over to talk with them. I told them that

I was a friend of Guiying's family. It turned out that they were all Guiying's neighbors and all of them knew about her mental illness. I did not mean to talk about Guiying's illness with her neighbors, but these villagers soon turned to this topic after Dong left.

A woman in her 30s said, "Guiying used to be normal, but after she had that illness, she began acting weird." Another one refuted, "That's not true, even before she went crazy, I had that feeling that she was abnormal. She talked a lot, but she could barely say one thing clearly."

An old lady stepped in and said, "She must have been possessed by someone. You know, her father-in-law died that night, and she did not go to take care of the dead old man. That is unfilial. She was supposed to be there with her family together. I guess the dead old man got angry at her and somehow possessed her." Several women seemed scared when they heard of this.

A middle-aged man laughed off this explanation, "That is nonsense. In my perspective, this is all about fate. She and her husband make lots of money all these years, and then their old man died, the wife went crazy, and their son was in a lawsuit. That sounds weird, but it does make sense if you consider this: you get something; you lose something, and then you have nothing left in the end. That is what life is about."

"Do you feel she becomes dangerous because of her mental illness?" I questioned.

"Of course, if you had been around that night when she went crazy, you would have known how dangerous she could be. We chased her around the village and tried to stop her. Finally when several strong young men pressed her to the ground and bound her with a strong rope, she was still shouting, singing and kicking." A woman said, posturing herself to show how those young men bound Guiying and how Guiying was shouting and kicking at the time.

"What about after she was hospitalized?"

"She walks around like she is always on a mission. Nobody knows what she is doing. Nobody really cares. Sometimes she starts to talk nonsense to nobody all of a sudden, which is really scary."

Another woman cut in and raised her voice, saying, "She is absolutely dangerous. A few days ago, I was working on something at home, while my son was playing right outside the door. Later I came out to check on my son and found out she was talking to my son by the door. I was so scared. I asked my son to get back to the house and then I shut the door."

"Did she do anything to your son?"

"She was talking to my son, I did not notice what else she was doing. But who knows what she would have done if I showed up a few minutes later. You never know." An old lady nodded, "That is true. Your son is too young; it is good always to be careful, juts in case. Who knows what she could do? She is crazy. Do not get too close to her."

"If there is a wedding or a funeral, would she be invited to come over?"

All women started to look at one another, one said, "Who dares to invite her? She is nuts! What if she went crazy on the scene? Sometimes we did ask her to come over when we happened to run into her, but we were just trying to be nice, she also knew that and never comes to these events."

"If a person became like her, she would be no longer a person. Nobody cares about what she thinks or how she feels." A woman sighed, and then added, "truly, it is painful to her, but there is nothing we can do. We have to take care of ourselves."

Half an hour later, I was sitting in Zhao's truck on my way back to downtown Jian'an. Zhao has been running freight transportation with his truck for years, which is a sideline in addition to farming. "It is not easy to make a living in today's rural areas. There is no hope at all if you are just farming. You have to do something else to make money. That is why most of the young people in our village leave home and go to da gong in the cities. If you have some connections, you can go to da gong in the big cities like Beijing, Shanghai and Guangzhou where you can make big money; if not, you can at least go to Jian'an to make a little money. Everyone has their own ways to make a living."

I tried to move the conversation back to Guiying. Zhao told me that he was one of those who helped calm down Guiying when she went crazy that night. I asked him about Guiying's being avoided, teased and disdained after she got sick. "It is always like that when you became a person like her. That does not surprise me at all. If they don't do so, I will be surprised."

"Do you think that is discrimination against her?"

"Discrimination? If you say so, then it is. We do not use that word. There is no such a sense in people's mind. But who cares? She is crazy. She does not even feel or think. Do you think somebody is going to care how she feels? No way."

"She is miserable and pathetic in that painful situation; at least she deserves some sympathy. What do you say?"

"She does not even feel, how could she feel she is pathetic? She knows nothing and feels nothing. The real pathetic ones are her family. They are pathetic because they have to see that she is teased and fooled. They can still feel and think, so they are really pathetic."

The truck lurched on the harsh countryside road. Zhao slowed down and continued, "You are talking about pathetic. But who else is not pathetic? I mean, in rural areas. You tell me. We wake up early in the morning and stay up till late at night. Whatever we are doing is trying to feed those mouths in our families."

"Well, that is true, but, come on, your situation is still much better than hers, and at least you can live a normal life." I refuted Zhao's point and then went on to joke, "at least you have a truck. That is really something."

Zhao laughed off my joke, saying, "Let me tell you something. You might think I can make big money by driving my truck. But things might not be what they look like. You have no idea how it is difficult for us, I mean farmers, to make a living in today's society. We are treated as secondary citizens everywhere. They can do whatever they want to us. Especially those traffic police officers, they stop my truck everywhere and ask for all kinds of certificates of which I have never heard. If I don't have them, there will be a fine of hundreds of yuan; otherwise they are going to tow away the truck. I have never seen them do the same to those cars owned by urban people. If we go to the city, they think we are poor, dirty, rude and senseless. They never treat us with any politeness. You just mentioned discrimination; I think that is discrimination against farmers by urban people. Anyway, if you are a farmer from rural areas, none treat you as someone. What can we do about it? We have little choice but to accept it."

Zhao's argument that all rural people are miserable, discriminated, and stigmatized cannot justify the way they treat the stigmatized like

Guiying, but it does demonstrate how they look at Guiying from their own perspectives. For Guiying, her illness and the suffering it caused are everything in her daily life; for those villagers who stigmatize Guiying, however, her illness and suffering are nothing important to the extent that they will take it as their own priority. They have their own pain and suffering that they have to face up to and take care of, which are what really matters to them in their own lives. Basically villagers tend to ignore Guiying's suffering and her personhood if she does not appear violent, but when Guiying poses a danger or threat to themselves and their own families, they will take on a radically stigmatizing stance and act.

Guiying's mental illness reduced her into a non-person by shutting down her social relations and social networks. Being a non-person, she has been disdained, teased and avoided; her fear results from the isolation caused by the shutdown of social relations and social networks; her feeling and social face are denied and unacknowledged; she is not invited to attend any family event anymore because her presence is regarded as improper and disfacing. Moreover, Guiying's internalization of stigma and her management of stigma further prevent her from re-establishing social relations and social networks. She tried to regain her identity and right to be a person because of her consideration of other's feeling and social face, which places her in a more solidly non-person situation from which she can never escape.

Stigma Within a Mental Hospital — Go Get Your Medicine; I Don't Have Time for This

Jiangxia, another city about one hundred kilometers to the southwest of Jian'an, is the second site of my research. Compared to Jian'an, Jiangxia looks undeveloped, with a small size of urban area surrounded by larger rural areas. This city has a mental hospital opening up since the 1950s, which, among the first several mental hospitals in China, have initially been established to treat traumatized soldiers back from the Korean War in the early 1950s.

The hospital was located far away from downtown and close to the rural area. The time I arrived at the hospital, despite the fact that the whole hospital looked like a forsaken old park, the building for inpatient services was being rebuilt. A four-floor building for outpatient clinics was placed next to the main entrance of the hospital. In the innermost space of the hospital yard was located a two-floor building for patients with most serious mental illnesses. It looked like a bunker with several small ironbound windows installed at the height that cannot be reached from the ground. I could not get into that building, "it is too dangerous," Dr. Xiao said. He was showing me around the hospital on my first day there.

I met Jiasheng at Dr. Xiao's outpatient clinic. Jiasheng, a farmer of 35 years old, has been suffering insomnia and unhappiness for all the years. Before he came to seek help from Dr. Xiao, he had been seeing doctors at several local general hospitals for his insomnia, where he was diagnosed with neurasthenia and given various medicines. However, as he said, his symptoms remained.

Dr. Xiao diagnosed Jiasheng's problem as depression. When Dr. Xiao started to write Jiasheng his prescription, Jiasheng went on to talk about his family problems. He was pale and looked very tired, with his eyes alternately downcast or glancing at Dr. Xiao and his right hand rubbing his chest. He murmured intermittently in a drained voice of someone in mourning.

Jiasheng's family has been undergoing serious financial problems. His wife had been sick for years and he, to quote his own words, "also has serious health problem and cannot take hard work." Despite the difficult family financial situation, the whole family appeared to still urge their lone daughter to finish high school and even move on to college, which often does not apply to many families in poor rural areas. In fact, many families ask their children to drop out of school and find a job to make money as soon as they can because of the huge burden and tremendous pressure caused by a difficult family financial situation.

"We do so in hope that she can attend college and find a better job rewarded by good salary. For farmers like us, the life is hopeless. There is no way out. But she has her own chance to end this and start a totally new life. Attending college might be the only way to get her out of this awkward situation and even change the future of her own children. I won't let whatever has happened to us happen again to her," Jiasheng said.

Unfortunately, things do not always work out as people hope. The girl failed the entrance exam to college. "It was like a bolt from the blue. There had been a thread of light, but all of a sudden, everything was in dark. I just felt the sky collapsed." Jiasheng beat his own chest with his right fist, appearing in pain. He used to hold the hope that his daughter's college dream could change their hopeless family situation. But now that dream did not come true, instead it remained a dream. Jiasheng said, "I felt I lost everything at that moment, my only hope is gone."

While Jiasheng was speaking about his family suffering, Dr. Xiao kept his head down, looking at the prescription and did not respond with a single word. After he finished the prescription, he handed it to Jiasheng, saying, "Go get your medicine," without any comment on Jiasheng's narrative.

Jiasheng held the prescription paper in his hands and read it stutteringly. He seemed to have no intention to leave right away. He continued to articulate his desperate feeling, saying, "I just cannot believe this is happening. Look at my family, what are we going to do? It will cost more money to have my daughter take the exam again in the following year, but what if she fails again. We don't even have that amount of money. What are we going to do?" Still no response from Dr. Xiao, he was sitting behind his desk, staring at a corner of the room, and did not even look at Jiasheng.

Apparently, Jiasheng wanted to have someone listen to his painful feeling stuck in his chest; moreover, he had something other than the symptoms of his illness to talk about. When Jiasheng noticed that Dr. Xiao was not interested in his family story at all, he stopped his narrative of suffering and turned to ask about the prescription while holding it in his hands. This time, Dr. Xiao finally responded to him but with only a few words. Jiasheng went on to ask about the medicine in detail. Dr. Xiao became impatient and kept interrupting him, saying, "That is it. Just do as I tell you. You don't have to know those things. It is complicated; I don't have to explain everything to you. I don't have time for this. By the way, you won't understand it even if I tell you, it is going to be a waste of time. That is it, ok? Go get your medicine."

The clinic was not busy at all at the time. Jiasheng was the only one on the waiting list. Dr. Xiao should have had time to speak to Jisheng, if he wanted; however, he was not interested in that conversation at all. But Jiasheng seemed really to need someone to talk to and listen to his family story. He asked Dr. Xiao about his medication, and then repeated his complains of insomnia, dizziness and lack of energy. Dr. Xiao interrupted him again and raised his voice, saying, "Go get your medicine first, ok?" Jiasheng stood up with a worn umbrella under his arm and the prescription paper in his hands. He walked out of the clinic in a quiet, slow manner.

After Jiasheng left the clinic room, I asked Dr. Xiao, "Is psychotherapy available at this hospital? I mean, is there anyone patients can talk to about something else other than the disease and symptoms?"

"We don't have staff working specifically on that issue. Sometimes we do that work ourselves if we got time. But medicine is the most important. Talk does not resolve any problem. Only medicine can control and relieve patient's symptoms. That is for sure. These people are farmers; they know nothing and can barely say one thing. You can hardly talk to them on anything seriously. They talked a lot, but most of what they said has nothing to do with the disease and treatment."

After picking up his medicine, Jiasheng did not leave; instead, he came back to the clinic room and sat down, facing to Dr. Xiao, as he did earlier. This time, he began to read the instruction attached to the medicine bottle and asked Dr. Xiao about it. Dr. Xiao did not give him a detailed explanation, remaining silent most of the time. After a while, Jiasheng went back to repeating his family suffering. In the end, his narrative came to be a cycle without end: from medications to symptoms, and on to poor family situation, going round and round. Only when Jiasheng asked about his medication (What is it? What is it for?), Dr. Xiao would give him a simple and short answer; otherwise he would not speak one word. When Jiasheng found that Dr. Xiao was not responding to his story, he would stop, and then proceed to ask the same questions about his medications he asked several minutes before. Accordingly, he received the same replies he received the last turn of this conversation cycle. Jiasheng kept repeating his narrative of symptoms and family story, despite that fact Dr. Xiao remained silent all the time. In this way, the doctor-patient conversation moved in repetitive cycles.

After a while Dr. Xiao asked Jiasheng to take an electrocardiogram in order to break Jiasheng's narrative cycle. After it was done, Jiasheng came back again. This time, he found out that the name of the medication on one of those medication bottles was different from the one Dr. Xiao wrote on the prescription. Then Jiasheng started to ask what the difference is and why they are different. Later Jiasheng continued to repeat his symptoms, already dead hope, and unbearable family situation. The cycle appeared again.

Clearly Jiasheng had a pressing need to have someone to get to know his "deep pain" in his heart, which, I believe, no medication could cure. Jiasheng was one of the most talkative patients I have met, but the impression I had from his narrative was that he was completely crushed by his suffering caused by long-term stress and sudden despair. The difficult family financial situation placed him in long-term stress; while his daughter's exam failure added the last straw and put him into a desperate situation. Eventually sudden despair following long-term stress overwhelmed him.

In the Chinese cultural tradition, the middle aged, especially men, have been placed in the most stressful situation within family because they have to take care of both their parents and children whom they are not supposed to complain to, no matter the stress resulting from their works or from within family. In addition, Chinese people, in general, consider speaking about family stress in front of people outside their families to be shameful and a loss of social face. Thus, most of them keep stress in their hearts and have never spoken out. Therefore, if a man starts to speak out about his suffering in front of others, it means he is no longer able to stand the stress by himself and is already overwhelmed.

When people are eventually overwhelmed by stress and have to go to see a doctor, medical professionals become the only ones they can talk to, while the hospital might be the only place where they can speak out the suffering stuck in their hearts. However, as I have observed in the field, few medical professionals pay attention to these narratives of suffering. Most are centered on treating disease with medicine in the scientific sense rather than dealing with illness experiences; they are giving medicine for controlling symptom, and they are not comforting a suffering soul.

Medical professionals, whom I observed or interviewed, assume that they do not stigmatize because they are the ones close to patients. They are working with patients and treating their diseases, how can they be the source of stigma? It seems that they are the only ones who are taking care of and concerned about psychotic patients. But it is for the very same reason that medical professionals are the only groups with access to patients' privacy and personal suffering, which makes their reaction of rejection and discrimination so effective at conveying stigma. The medical system might be the first place where patients' privacy is exposed. It is also the first place where patients perceive being stigmatized.

Stigma Within the Family — You Are Feigning Illness

I met Xiaojun at the Inpatient Department of Jiangxia Mental Hospital. He was 29 years old at the time, short and chubby. Thirteen years before, when he was taking the college entrance exam, he became psychotic for the first time. After that he has been hospitalized intermittently. In 2005, he was again hospitalized.

Xiaojun used to attend a local high school where his father was teaching. Later, on his own request, Xiaojun was transferred to another high school because he often had fights with his classmates. I also met Xiaojun's father, Mr. Chu, who was accompanying Xiaojun during his hospitalization, and we had many talks. In the course of these talks I learned that Mr. Chu had been very strict with Xiaojun and held a very high expectation for him. Xiaojun has a younger brother who used to study in Hunan University and then went to Tsinghua University for a master's degree. Chu was so proud of his younger son that he appeared very prideful every time when he mentioned the young man during our talks. At the moment I had the impression that the old man's pride came out of not only being a father but also being a high school teacher. It seemed that he considered his younger son to be a successful product of his professional career as being a teacher rather than a product of him being a father.

In my perspective, both the old man's high expectation and the younger brother's outstanding school performance placed Xiaojun into an extremely stressful situation and had a great impact on the onset of his illness.

Mr. Chu believes the fight that Xiaojun once had with several classmates caused Xiaojun's illness. After that fight, Xiaojun became hesitant to attend school; even when he was sitting in classroom, he was unable to concentrate on his study. Sometimes he took the bus to the suburbs and found a place to read the Bible. When Mr. Chu heard this from Xiaojun's teacher, he made a visit to Xiaojun's school. That day Mr. Chu found out that Xiaojun was wandering around alone on the school's playground during the class meeting time. Mr. Chu decided to bring Xiaojun back to the school where he was teaching and put Xiaojun under his own supervision. He criticized Xiaojun for not attending school, and asked him not to fantasize but study hard and look up to his younger brother.

But Mr. Chu's supervision did not work either; Xiaojun still could not concentrate on his study. Moreover, he began acting abnormal. At the end of September 1992, Mr. Chu accompanied Xiaojun to another province to visit a mental hospital. Owing to the strong stigma associated with mental illnesses, families are fearful that the mental illness within the family could be exposed in public; they generally tend to hide this situation from local people and send the mentally ill family members to remote places for diagnoses and hospitalization. This also applied to Xiaojun's case. As Mr. Chu recalled, doctors informed them that they could give Xiaojun treatments, but the bad news was that Xiaojun could never be cured. Those doctors didn't even tell Mr. Chu and Xiaojun the diagnosis, thus they had no idea what kind of specific mental illness Xiaojun had. Nonetheless, Xiaojun was hospitalized there.

Xiaojun's younger brother, who was studying at Hunan University at the time, heard this news and immediately came to take Xiaojun out of the hospital and bring him back home. Xiaojun's brother did not believe Xiaojun had a mental illness; he even blamed his father for sending Xiaojun to a mental hospital. He was fearful that the stigma associated with mental illness would destroy the life chances of his older brother. He blamed his father, "Are you out of your mind? How could he have a mental illness? You are not saving him but destroying his life." Mr. Chu recalled this instance, saying, "He was worried about Xiaojun at the time. I understand that. They were close to each other. Now when I think back, I felt he just could not accept the fact that Xiaojun had a mental illness. Another thing he was afraid of is the stigma that comes with mental illness. But who else in the family would like to accept that?"

Xiaojun's problem remained, though his younger brother refused to admit it. About the time Xiaojun's mental illness became too prominent to be hidden from others; he was hospitalized again at a local hospital. This time there was no need to hide the situation and send Xiaojun away because everyone in the neighborhood already knew about Xiaojun's mental illness. The whole family still suspected if Xiaojun really had a mental illness. They were still holding hope, however, that Xiaojun could have been misdiagnosed in the first place. After Spring Festival in 1994, Xiaojun, accompanied by his father, went to Hunan Mental Hospital (Changsha, the capital of Hunan Province) for a final diagnosis. Subsequently, Xiaojun was diagnosed with schizophrenia.

I talked to Xiaojun several times. He attributed his mental illness to his overconfident personality. Another day he told me that the major cause of his school failure was lack of motivation to enter college. "I dedicated myself to study because I wanted to honor my family by attending college," Xiaojun said, "that used to be the major factor that motivated me to study hard. But my brother had been very successful in school and already attended university. In that sense, he has already made enough social face for our family, thus I don't have that motivation any more. It was like the family mission that we had taken on all those years had been accomplished. There was no need to do it again. Therefore, school no longer matters to me." I prefer to believe that Xiaojun was using this reason, lack of motivation, as a pretext to disguise his mental collapse under the great impact brought by the family's high expectation for him and his brother's success.

Xiaojun was not allowed to attend the college entrance exam because of his mental illness, so ended his school life. Later Mr. Chu found him a job at the local revenue bureau. Soon his work mates found out that Xiaojun was abnormal, and then, in a few days, he lost the job. After that Xiaojun worked at his father's school as a doorman. In 2001, Xiaojun became very asocial and would not leave home. He often repeats to himself "don't worry, don't worry" dozens of times before he leaves home, and "I will be better, I will be better" more than fifty times before he goes to bed at nights.

Xiaojun and his father both acknowledged that, in general, there was a strong stigma against people who have mental illness. His father said that stigma is caused by people's lack of knowledge about mental illness and the absence of social support networks for patients. His speech did not surprise me because I learned from my conversations with him that he had read books related to mental illness ever since Xiaojun was diagnosed with schizophrenia. Mr. Chu always speaks the way that he would in his classroom; he speaks as if he is reading textbook. However, Mr. Chu denied that stigma exists in Xiaojun's case. He said, "Most people in our neighborhood are concerned about Xiaojun; a few people sometimes tease him. You know, that happens sometimes. But there is no such thing as discrimination or stigma ever happening to him. Right now, the most important thing is to help him to get on with his life as soon as possible. He is already 29 years old. It is time for him to get married and make his own family."

I believe that most patients and their families do not like to tell others that they are suffering great social stigma even if they really are because of the issue of social face. They are trying to save their own faces by denying or disguising the stigma. When you get very familiar with patients and their families, they might tell the truth; but the reality is that people usually tend to disguise their suffering caused by stigma and are reluctant to admit that they are stigmatized. In general, people tend to say that "stigma does exist, but it does not happen to me". The denial of stigma, as a stigma management technique, once again indicates that the issue of social face is closely related to stigma: the operating mechanism of stigma is to undermine social face by identifying the stigmatized as a non-person; while the stigmatized try to save social face by denying that they are stigmatized. No matter if it works, denying and disguising might be the last hope the stigmatized can hold on to in order to maintain their rights and dignity.

A most dramatic event happened when one afternoon I was talking to Xiaojun and his father. Mr. Chu's younger sister and her husband, a cadre working for the local government, showed up at the ward to check on Xiaojun's condition. The minute he walked into the ward, the cadre started to criticize Xiaojun, "Look at you, so feckless! You don't even look like a person! Do you have any idea what you are doing? You don't have any illness; I know that, you are just too lazy. In the past, you did not go to school because you did not want to study; now you don't want to work, you are just lazy. You don't have any illness; I know you are feigning illness. I tell you, there is no such illness at all." The cadre shouted at Xiaojun, standing in the center of the ward with his hands behind his back.

Xiaojun started to sob with tears trickling down his chin. Mr. Chu's eyes were also full of tears. The stern cadre continued, "What are you crying for? Do you have any idea how busy we are? We have work to do every day, but now we have to find time to come over to see you? It is a waste of time! You see how many people are here for you? You don't deserve this!" And then the cadre stopped and looked at me, "This is our family matter, will you just leave us?" I had to leave. The cadre slammed the door behind me. I heard that the cadre continued to complain, "This is a family matter, ok? Don't talk to anyone outside! Do you think this is some honor you can show around and tell everyone? What a shame! ..." It seemed to me that Xiaojun's uncle, owing to his social status, considered himself the real leader in this family and assume that he has the responsibility to correct the entire family's misunderstanding of Xiaojun's illness.

Xiaojun's brother refused to admit that Xiaojun had a mental illness because of his fear of stigma related to mental illness. Mr. Chu denied that Xiaojun had been stigmatized in order to save face for Xiaojun and the entire family. The cadre, also Xiaojun's uncle, criticized Xiaojun for feigning illness. He resisted acknowledging Xiaojun's mental illness as a real illness, and considered it family shame. Feigning illness is an excuse meant to normalize and repel stigma, but in fact it demonstrates how powerful stigma is.

All of these reactions confirm that there is severe stigma associated with mental illness; it has close relations with the issue of social face; whatever stigma means for people has much to do with what it is like to be a person in the local life world. This case also indicates that stigma exists within the family, not just in work units, local communities and medical institutions. The family is also a place where its members with mental illness can be stigmatized. Compared to other stigmatizing sites, the family plays a more significant role when it comes to deepen operating mechanism of stigma, because the family features a tight social space, intimate relationships and frequent daily interactions, which promise intensive time for interpersonal experiences to express and amply stigma.

In this regard other stigmatizing sites are incomparable. What happens to the whole family and each of the members when one of them develops mental illness is clear to a degree hardly visible in other sites like the work unit, local community, and medical institution.

Summary

The cases I included in this chapter show that people with mental illness are stigmatized in work unit, village, hospital and family. Jianguo was teased in his work unit mainly because of his unsocial personality. He was considered a non-person without dignity. Guiying's mental illness was connected to her family history of rise and fall and involved with her father-in-law's death and her son's being arrested. She was perceived as a threat to public safety in the village and considered a non-person who was unable to feel how normal person feel and did not deserve sympathy. Jiasheng felt hopeless after his daughter failed to enter college, which he thought was the last hope for the entire family. He was considered a problematic patient who always complained a lot. Xiaojun was blamed by his uncle for pretending to be sick. Wen's case suggested that people with psychosis was stigmatized and treated as non-persons even among the mentally ill persons.

In the case of mental illness, stigma has much to do with what makes a person in the local world, which is related to the issue of social face, social relationships, and social networks in the Chinese context. On the stigmatized side, stigma results from lack of social face caused by the absence of social relations and social networks; on the stigmatizer side, people stigmatize someone because they consider the person a non-person who is unable to be a person and therefore does not deserve to be treated as a normal person with social face and dignity. By treating a person with disrespect, people also protect and amplify their own social and moral status.

Mental illness reduces a person to a non-person by shutting down the patient's social relationships and social networks. A non-person is disdained, teased and avoided; his/her feeling and social face are denied and unacknowledged. In the local world, the stigmatized's illness and suffering are not important to the extent that other people will take it as their own priority; rather, they have their own priority to take care of, which is what really matters to them in their own lives. People tend to ignore the stigmatized if they do not appear violent. When people perceive the stigmatized becoming a threat to what matters most in their own lives, they will take on radically stigmatizing stance and act.

Stigma also exists among the stigmatized. In general, people with mental illness refuse to acknowledge that they have mental illness, and then deny that they are stigmatized, in part because of the shame caused by the internalization of stigma, or because of the management of stigma (by saving social face). The internalization of stigma and the management of stigma are both likely to lead to a further shutdown of social relations and social networks.

Work units, local communities, medical institutions, and families are major sites where people with mental illness are stigmatized. The family, as a mini society, provides a location where it is extremely clear to see how stigma operates in the local life world.

Chapter Three

Ethnography of stigma associated with HIV/AIDS in Beijing

Beijing

In March 2006, I moved to Beijing, the capital of China, and started conducting field research on stigma associated with HIV/AIDS. At the time, there was a prominent self-help program organized and managed by HIV/AIDS patients in Beijing. I once talked to the director of this program on telephone to see if they could give me the permission to conduct my research there. But I was refused, and then I went on to tell them that I could work for them as a volunteer while doing my research. The director said, "We don't need any volunteer. Yes, we have hundreds of volunteers registered on board, but we never really need their help. In fact, we have never contacted them." I knew that without any personal connection I would not be accepted by these HIV/AIDS groups because they build a wall around themselves in order to limit the impact of strong stigma associated with HIV/AIDS, but I still wanted to give it a try to see how strong the stigma is. The next week I used some connections to find another AIDS care organization, AIDS Care Center, and was accepted. Later during my stay in Beijing, and through AIDS Care Center where I worked, I found a way to get to know the organization that turned me down.

AIDS Care Center in Beijing

AIDS Care Center, an NGO, was established in 2001 and has been providing medical information, support care, family intervention and legal consultation for HIV/AIDS patients, and also developing HIV/AIDS prevention programs among MSM (men have sex with men) groups. Its office was located at the Fourth People's Hospital, a hospital featuring treating infectious diseases in Beijing; the Center has been working closely with the STD Clinic of this hospital. According to the official statistics from the Fourth People's Hospital, the STD Clinic had received more than 3,000 cases of HIV/AIDS by the beginning of 2006. Of the patients who had residency permit in Beijing more than 90% were gay men, while the rest claimed they were infected through tainted blood transfusion or sexual intercourse.

AIDS Care Center has benefited from its official affiliation with the Fourth People's Hospital. Since it's very beginning the Center has been receiving financial and technical support from the government through the hospital. Because of these facts, other NGOs working on HIV/AIDS who generally have difficulty in accessing resources and support from the government often question the validity of AIDS Care Center's NGO identity.[1] In 2006, the regular staff of the Center included: a director, Ding, the former nurse-in-chief from the STD Clinic, and several patient volunteers of whom Zhanshan had been working for years on HIV/AIDS care consulting: including hotline, crisis intervention, and partner education and care. Ding was a middle-aged lady with great patience for her daily work; she welcomed me to work as both a volunteer and a researcher at the Center. Although Ding was really nice to me, it did not make my first several days at the Center easier. On my first day at the Center Ding

[1] In today's China, the NGOs basically have two major funding sources: government or international foundations, in addition to a small amount of individual donations. Among the NGOs, a few of them that are acknowledged and supported by the government like AIDS Care Center in Beijing are called official NGOs who have all supports (financial support, technical support, and more important, official cooperation) needed to manage and develop projects, while other NGOs often find it difficult to start up or develop due to lack of official acknowledgment and cooperation from the governments at all levels, though they sometimes get large amounts of money from international foundations.

introduced Zhanshan and me to each other; we both said hello. After that, Zhanshan would not talk to me anymore. I decided to wait, not to be aggressive and posing questions in the beginning.

During the first several days at the Center, I temporarily put my research aside and focused on volunteer work: receiving patients, doing paper work, helping them move around various stuff, such as health education booklets, magazines called *Friends* aimed at gay men groups and *Hand in Hand* published for HIV/AIDS patients, mailing medicine to patients living in other provinces, and picking up boxes of condoms from CDC that were going to be distributed among gay men groups for the sake of safe sex. During my stay at the AIDS Care Center, I had been working at the Center as a volunteer while doing my research. Generally, Mrs. Ding would introduce me to patients and the other clinic staff as a volunteer; but they also knew that I was conducting a research at the Center.

Zhanshan

As time went on, I noticed that several patients visited AIDS Care Center a lot and they often came in without any specific reason. Zhanshan seemed to be a leader of this group of HIV/AIDS patients: Every patient was happy to see him, loved to talk to him, and treated him as if he were their oldest brother; while Zhanshan also treated other patients as brothers and sisters. Zhanshan and I got to know each other better; we even took cigarette breaks together on the patio outside of the STD Clinic, behind us there was a No Smoking sign on the wall. Zhanshan was a heavy smoker and consumed at least two packs of cigarettes a day, which is not good for his health especially in terms of his AIDS situation. But nobody could have persuaded him to quit smoking. He once told me, "Cigarettes are like food to me. How can I survive without food?"

Zhanshan gradually became interested in my research and started asking about it; I also asked him about his family, but not at the very beginning about his illness experience. Zhanshan even showed me photos of his family, including his father and lovely daughter. One day, Zhanshan told me that I was different from other volunteers he had met before. "You are not like them." Zhanshan smiled at me, "a lot of volunteers came and left from time to time, but most of them were just curious about how we, HIV/AIDS patients, look. They came here like they were visiting a zoo to see an exotic animal and kept asking us all kinds of stupid, naïve questions. When they finally found out we do not look that different from anyone they could meet on the streets, they were no longer interested in staying with us." Eventually I figured out why the self-help group of HIV/AIDS patients I contacted first turned me down. They thought I was one of those "naïve" volunteers who have nothing but curiosity. I took Zhanshan's words as a sign of acceptance. Later we became close friends.

Zhanshan was 48 years old and living with his father and daughter. I once asked Zhanshan about his wife. "We got divorced after I got HIV. It was not her idea; I suggested that we should get divorced, and then she agreed. There is no need to waste her time. I am finished, but she is still young." Zhanshan stopped, looking down at the cigarette burning between his fingers, and then went on, "She is a nice person; we still talk to each other on telephone. Sometimes we get together for a meal."

"Did your daughter know of your disease?"

"I don't know. I didn't tell her. But I always leave my medications around my apartment and never hide them from her. My daughter is a smart girl. So I guess she might already know it. But we have never talked about it." A gentle smile came over Zhanshan's face when he spoke of his daughter.

Zhanshan was born into an ordinary family in Beijing in the 1950s. During the Cultural Revolution (1966–1976), he went to a village in Hebei to "receive re-education from poor peasants" as hundreds of thousands youth of his age did at the time. By the end of Cultural Revolution, owing to lack of connection, Zhanshan had no choice but to bribe the rural cadres to get out of the village. After he returned to Beijing, he found a job at a state-run bakeshop and started his career as a worker.

In 2000, Zhanshan felt a pain within his chest. He went to see a doctor at a general hospital, and then he was diagnosed with tuberculosis and hospitalized. Soon doctors found out that Zhanshan had a symptom of persistent high fever that generally is not supposed to occur in the case of tuberculosis. Therefore, they took Zhanshan's blood sample without telling him about the purpose, an HIV test.

In the following several days, having not heard anything about his blood test, Zhanshan became nervous. One day, he was not feeling well and asked nurses for help, but none showed up; instead, when Zhanshan stepped out of his wardroom for help, all nurses rushed into nurse's station room and locked themselves inside. As Zhanshan went over, a nurse shouted at him behind the door, "Do you have any idea what kind of disease you have? You freak! Go away and be quiet!!" Zhanshan was totally lost. He had no idea what was going on, but he sensed that his blood test went wrong and he might have had some unusual disease.

The next day when Zhanshan was wandering in the lobby, a young nurse came up at a distance, saying, "Please go back to your room, or I am going to lose my job. Please!" The young nurse appeared shaken when she was speaking. Zhanshan had to do as she suggested, though he did not know why. But right after he entered his wardroom, the nurse immediately shut and locked the door behind him and then ran away. As Zhanshan found out that all of his ward beddings were gone, he became extremely angry; but what he could do was just shouting at nobody in his locked wardroom. Then someone standing outside the door shouted back at him, "What are you shouting for? You people deserve this! Be quiet!" A few days later Zhanshan's father and sister showed up at his wardroom, they told Zhanshan that they were informed by the hospital that Zhanshan had to be transferred to another hospital. Zhanshan's sister did not tell him outright but hinted that he had AIDS according to his blood test result. Zhanshan eventually figured out why those nurses had been treating him that way over those days. All of a sudden, he felt his head is blank.

"My sister was speaking to me, but I could barely hear one word. I felt that sweat kept coming down from my head and my shirt was soaked by sweat in a few minutes. Later I put myself together and made a decision. I asked my sister if she had money. She gave me 2,000 yuan. I took it and then wanted to leave. My father and sister tried to stop me, but I just walked away; I didn't even look back. At the moment I just felt I had to leave, though I had no idea where to go. I guess I just wanted to go away." That day, Zhanshan took a long walk without destination till late night. "Walking alone in the dark at night, you don't know where you are heading or what is ahead of you. That is how this disease makes you feel," added Zhanshan.

Zhanshan and I were having this conversation on a cigarette break. He had another puff at his cigarette, and then went on in a slow and sad manner, "Over these years, I just don't understand why they (medical staffs) treated me that way in the first place. They are doctors and nurses, and they have professional medical knowledge. They should have known better about this disease than ordinary people. Why did they act the same way as ordinary people did? That was a nightmare. I did not know what to do or what to think. I thought about suicide, but later I told myself that I have to survive no matter what happened. In fact, suicide is a much easier choice than struggling to survive; you simply need more courage to live on than giving up and kill yourself. I was dying when I was hospitalized at this hospital (the Fourth People's Hospital) for the first time. But finally I survived." Zhanshan took a deep breath and then continued, "I knew I might have had AIDS some day because I am a gay. But before that day I thought it was a foreign disease that did not exist in China."

The first HIV/AIDS case in China was documented in 1985. The patient was an Argentine-American tourist who died of AIDS at Xiehe (Peking union) Hospital in Beijing. In the following several years, the Infectious Diseases Prevention Center tested 310 blood samples collected across the country among hemophilia patients who had used imported blood product, especially factor VIII. It turned out that three of them were HIV positive. In addition, an international student from Congo was found HIV positive. In 1987, another HIV case was found in Fujian province. The patient was a native but had been living in Hong Kong and the United States over ten years before he returned to China for medical help. In China before the 1990s, HIV/AIDS had been deemed as a foreign (capitalistic) disease that did not exist in a socialistic society like China. "The corrupted western bourgeoisie life style" was believed to have provided the hotbed for all social evils, such as prostitution, drug use, and homosexuality, which resulted in various diseases including HIV/AIDS. At the time, the Chinese government asserted that the absence of HIV/AIDS in socialistic China constituted substantial evidence of the superiority of socialism over capitalism.

In 1985, the Ministry of Health submitted a report (*weibaofangzi*, No. 78, 1985) to the State Council, remarking that sexual intercourse is a major HIV infection route and calling on medical system to monitor the health condition of foreigners who were traveling in China and prostitutes who have sex with foreigners. At the end of the report, the Ministry of Health asked the Ministry of Treasury for financial support to import medical equipment needed in order to deal with the HIV/AIDS epidemic. In 1986, the Ministry of Health issued a notice on strengthening national surveillance over HIV/AIDS epidemic (*weifangzi*, No. 1, 1986) and urged governments at all levels to take strong control over the information related to HIV/AIDS in order to keep people from panic and "bad influences". In 1987, the Ministry of Health submitted another report (*weibaofangzi*, No. 30, 1987) to the State Council and pointed out that there were four major sources of HIV infection in China: (1) foreigners; (2) prostitutes and gay men, (3) imported blood products, and (4) overlapping infection within hospitals due to the repetitive use of needles and surgery instruments. In this report, the Ministry of Health suggested that the Ministry of Public Security takes serious actions to crack down on underground prostitution. It stated, "Recently, owing to the influence of the corrupted capitalistic thoughts and life style, prostitution is spreading across the country, more and more people are infected with venereal diseases. Especially, a minority of prostitutes like to hang out and sleep with foreigners. Moreover, a number of gay men are also found in Tianjin and Haerbin. Even Hong Kong newspapers named Guangzhou a paradise of gay men."

The relevant laws and rules issued in China during the 1980s include the following.

1. 1985, Notice on Prohibition of the Importation of Blood Products (Factor VIII). (*weiyaozi*, No. 49, 1985).[2] It states, "Currently, the AIDS epidemic is spreading in the United States and Western Europe. By June 1984, more than 5,000 cases of AIDS had been found in the United States and the mortality among AIDS patients was up to 70–80%. According to the information reported from these countries, many people who have hemophilia and other diseases are infected by HIV through blood

[2]Co-issued by the Ministry of Health, the Ministry of economy and trade, and Main Customs Administration in 1985.

transfusion and other blood products, such as factor VIII. This suggests that using these blood products might cause AIDS. Since our country has not set up an effective HIV test system, it is risky to continue importation of blood products from foreign countries. In order to protect people's health and keep AIDS out of our country, we demand that no unit be allowed to import blood products from now on, including human plasma (frozen, liquid and freeze-dried), human normal immunoglobulin, immunoglobulin for intravenous administration, cryoprecipitated factor VIII, factor VIII concentrate, factor IX concentrate and prothrombin complex concentrate."

2. 1985, Law of the People's Republic of China on Control of the Entry and Exit of Aliens.[3] Article 12, aliens who are considered as a possible threat to China's state security and public order shall not be permitted to enter China.

3. 1986, Rules Governing the Implementation of the Law of the PRC on the Entry and Exit of Aliens.[4] Article 7, aliens coming under the following categories shall not be allowed to enter China: (1) An alien expelled by the Chinese government and before the expiry of the period when his/her re-entry is prohibited; (2) An alien considered likely to engage in terrorism, violence or subversion upon entering China; (3) An alien considered likely to engage in smuggling, drug trafficking or prostitution upon entering China; (4) An alien suffering from mental disorder, leprosy, AIDS, venereal diseases, contagious tuberculosis or other infectious diseases;

---

[3]Adopted at the 13th Meeting of the Standing Committee of the Sixth National People's Congress, promulgated by Order No. 31 of the President of the People's Republic of China on November 22, 1985, and effective as of February 1, 1986. The English translation is compiled by the Bureau of Legislative Affairs of the State Council of the People's Republic of China, and is published by the China Legal System Publishing House in July 1991.

[4]Approved by the State Council on 3 December 1986 and Promulgated by the Ministry of Public Security and the Ministry of Foreign Affairs on 27 November 1986. Revised and Approved by the State Council on 13 July 1994 and Promulgated by the Ministry of Public Security and the Ministry of Foreign Affairs on 15 July 1994. The English translation is compiled by the Bureau of Legislative Affairs of the State Council of the People's Republic of China, and is published by the China Legal System Publishing House in July 1991.

(5) An alien who cannot guarantee to cover his/her own expenses during his/her stay in China; (6) An alien considered likely to engage in other activities prejudicial to China's national security and interests.

4. 1986, Notice on HIV test among international students (*jiaowaizongzi*, No. 676, 1986).[5] It demands that all international students, scholars and researchers take HIV test under the surveillance of universities and local health bureaus within one month after they enter China.

5. 1987, Rules Concerning Health Certification of Aliens on the Entry (*wenyijianzi*, No. 48, 1987).[6] It states that all foreigners entering China shall present health certification and take health tests, including tests for bubonic plague, cholera, yellow fever, venereal diseases, leprosy, contagious tuberculosis, AIDS, and mental disorders.

Epidemiology, directed by political ideology at the time, had come to dominate the Chinese government's policies to deal with the early epidemic of HIV/AIDS. Based on the idea that HIV/AIDS originates in foreign countries, the government's policies were mainly aimed to prevent it from entering China. All of these policies and related practices also reinforced the impression already formed among the general Chinese population that HIV/AIDS is a foreign disease that does not exist in China. Under this circumstance, it is understandable that those nurses in Zhanshan's case acted out of fear, panic and anger when they found out that a Chinese, not a foreigner, was HIV positive. It would be a shock. For that reason, it makes sense that the Chinese government had responded to the epidemic of HIV/AIDS — a threat and danger approaching from the outside capitalistic world — by denial, panic and concealment. As facts began conflicting with political ideology and propaganda they had long believed in, the spread of HIV/AIDS within China disgraced the Chinese government.

All of this makes Zhanshan's experiences more understandable. He seemed relaxed when we put his horrible memories behind and started talking about his current life. As I, an observer from outside, could tell,

[5] Co-issued by the ministry of Health and National Education Committee on 26 November 1986.

[6] Co-issued by the Ministry of Health and the Ministry of Public Security on 14 May 1987.

Zhanshan really enjoyed his work at the AIDS Care Center. He always seemed to be in high spirits whenever he talked to medical staffs or other patients. He had never missed a chance to tell jokes and be funny. Ding gave Zhanshan a highly positive evaluation on his work at the Center. She said, "He has been very dedicated to his work. We are lucky that we have him work with us. He has made a very important contribution to this program. There is no doubt that we could not have accomplished projects without his valuable help and effort."

It seemed to me that Zhanshan and other patients had established and maintained very good relations with all the medical staffs at the STD Clinic. There was no sign of stigma at all, if I just observed how they reacted to each other every day. I once asked Zhanshan about the issue of stigma. He replied, "You won't see stigma here because we have been working together for a long time. Some of us have been together for many years since the first day I was hospitalized at this hospital. We already got very familiar with all doctors and nurses. There is no stigma here, but if you go to other general hospitals, things are going to be quite different."

I also talked to Dr. Meng, the director of the STD Clinic, about stigma associated with HIV/AIDS within medical institutions. He admitted that it was a problem. In his perspective, people always assume that medical professionals know more about HIV/AIDS than ordinary people, but that might not be true, especially when it comes to general hospitals. "Those medical professionals at general hospitals generally know little, if not nothing, about HIV/AIDS. They are as afraid of HIV/AIDS as ordinary people are. When our patients go to see them for opportunistic infections,[7] they became scared once they hear the word HIV/AIDS. In the case of HIV/AIDS, many medical professionals are not as knowledgeable as we expected. They do not know what to do either. Basically, stigma is caused by people's ignorance and misunderstanding of HIV/AIDS. People don't

[7] Opportunistic infection, it occurs frequently in a weak immune system. HIV attacks and weakens immune system, which provides an opportunity for various antigens to infect. In general, compared to the healthy people, HIV/AIDS patients are likely to get more infections and develop more critical diseases because of their compromised immune system.

know what kind of disease it is, so they don't know how to deal with it. That's why they are so afraid of it."

"Stigma is also related to the professional attitude of medical workers. We also had this problem at this clinic, though we have been specifically treating this disease for many years." Dr. Meng went on to tell me a story, "A few months ago, we conducted a questionnaire survey on stigma among HIV/AIDS patients we have treated at our clinic. The survey result really shocked me. It indicates that patients regarded us, medical professionals, as the source of stigma. It did not make any sense to me at all in the first place. I thought we are the ones who are treating and helping these patients, how could they refer to us as the ones who stigmatize and discriminate against them? Later I found out that many patients are not satisfied with the way we speak to them. I think sometimes we did unintentionally hurt their feelings. Sometimes we ignored how they feel, though we are treating these patients for their own good. You know this thing happens a lot in daily life. As a common saying puts it, 'the speaker speaks unintentionally, but the listener listens intentionally.' After that survey we have been working hard to improve our professional attitude. We have provided a lot of training to our staffs, and things are getting better. You know, it is not good enough to know you are doing the right thing; you have to know how to do it in the right way. In the past we had no idea about this, we just dealt with diseases, we thought that's our job, but now things have changed, people have higher expectations for us."

Dr. Meng soon turned away from his view of professional attitude, "But, in the face of HIV/AIDS epidemic, there are more important issues than stigma that we should put at the top of our priorities, such as dealing with opportunistic infections, providing HAART treatment, and improving prevention interventions.[8] If we have the effective medications that are able to kill all of those viruses and the effective vaccines that can keep all people safe from this epidemic, there will be no stigma because in that case HIV/AIDS will no longer be a deadly disease. Image one day HIV/AIDS comes to be a common disease like a curable STD or even a

[8]HAART, Highly Active Anti-Retroviral Therapy for HIV/AIDS, which generally combines several classes (protease inhibitor, integrase inhibitor, entry inhibitor, and maturation inhibitor) of antiretroviral drugs.

common disease like cold, how could people still be afraid of it? Thus, medication is definitely the final solution not only to the disease but also to the issue of stigma. Medicine should be the key we are holding to resolve all of these problems."

Doctors like Dr. Meng and many patients who have HIV/AIDS believe that, one day in the future, medication and vaccine that can turn HIV/AIDS into a curable and preventable disease are going to resolve all problems caused by this disease, including the disease itself and stigma resulting from it. On the medical professionals side, they believe so because of their belief in the power of medicine that they have witnessed over the course of the development of biomedicine; on patients side, stigma associated with HIV/AIDS is so strong that they can do nothing about it, while medication becomes their last hope that they can expect to change the whole painful situation by removing the disease from their bodies, and after that they will become a normal person as they once were. However, the current reality is that HIV/AIDS remains a chronic and deadly disease, treatable but incurable, despite all efforts to date dedicated to producing effective medicine and vaccine. Accordingly, stigma associated with HIV/AIDS remains a serious source of suffering that patients cannot simply ignore but have to face up to every day.

My argument is that stigma will never vanish even if HIV/AIDS is curable one day in the future; instead, it will always find the next or other vehicles to convey the same meaning as it does to the people who live with HIV/AIDS. There are always incurable diseases and unalleviated pain, no matter which period of human history you are living in. People who are living with HIV/AIDS today are only one of those countless vehicles for stigma. An effective medication or vaccine that can cure or prevent HIV/AIDS might remove stigma from the people who are living with HIV/AIDS, but they will never make stigma itself disappear because they do not work on the social genesis and operating mechanism of stigma. My concern is how these patients who have HIV/AIDS understand and respond to stigma associated with HIV/AIDS in their time.

Zhanshan clearly made his point on this issue to me as well as to many patients who came to him for help. He always put it this way, "We have this disease because of our own faults. We have none but ourselves to blame for this disease. If you get it, you have to deal with it no matter what it is going to cost you. You have to stand the psychical pain, stigma and social discrimination caused by the disease. Because you did something wrong in the past and you should have avoided what happened to you, you have to take it on your own. You have no right to ask others to treat you in a better way. You have no right to complain about being discriminated against. But that does not mean that you have to lock yourself at home, you can still try to live with a positive spirit in an active way. You just cannot expect something from others while doing nothing." Sometimes, Zhanshan became very angry with those patients who complained a lot. "Don't tell me that you are innocent. Don't cast yourself as someone innocent who does not deserve this. I am one of your people. We both know what we did before." Zhansha always said so when he could not stand other patients' complaints any more.

At first, I regarded Zhanshan's angry speech as embodiment of his self-stigmatization; however, later I found out that Zhanshan's self-criticism has more to do with something else. One Friday, Zhanshan invited me and two other patients, his best patient friends, Xiulan and her husband, to have dinner together. After work we went to a restaurant. We sat down and ordered some food and beer, and then we started eating, drinking, and talking. Things did not go unusual until Zhanshan suddenly burst into sobs after several bottles of beer. Before that day, he always looked happy and satisfied with his work; but that night he complained about his feeling of unfairness in his work experience at AIDS Care Center. "I have done so much work for the Center, but I still feel I am someone outside of it. They have never treated me as an official staff but a patient volunteer," Zhanshan's eyes brimmed with tears, and his hand holding a beer bottle appeared shaken, "and they have never given me any official position or title. Every time I go to attend conferences, all of those patients working for other organizations exchange their cards with each other, but I don't have anything, I have nothing to bring out. I am even afraid to tell other people that I am working for the Center because I don't have any certificate for that. I am not asking for these things, it is about the way I have been treated, which makes me feel that I don't belong to this Center. They might think that because they let me work for them, that itself is some kind of gracious gift, thus I should not ask for more than that. It is like that I, as a patient, already got enough and should not demand more than what I was given." Zhanshan's complaint would never make sense to me if I just observed how he was doing at the Center. At the moment, I was a little shocked and did not know what to say but tried to comfort him, saying, "Everybody know what you have been doing. They always appreciate your great help." Xiulan also tried to calm Zhanshan, "We all know that. Ding also knows of it, but there is nothing more she can do about it. You should know that some institutional affairs are far beyond her control." Zhanshan replied, "I just feel my work has never been acknowledged, officially. That is the reason I feel I have not been treated fairly enough."

To understand Zhanshan's complaint, we have to take the background of the AIDS Care Center into consideration. The AIDS Care Center is registered as an NGO, but it is officially operated by the Fourth People's Hospital. Even though Ding is the director of this NGO, she remains an official staff of the hospital from which she has been receiving her salary; while Zhanshan, as a patient volunteer, does not have any official affiliation with the hospital, receiving about 500 yuan from his hotline consulting program funded by a foundation. In China, a lot of HIV/AIDS patients lost their job when their work units found out about their AIDS status. Although the work units run by the state are not allowed to fire their staff, they generally deprive these patients of their work positions, remove them from their offices, and suggest that they do not work anymore. Even if these patients still receive salary from their work units, they often have difficulty in getting reimbursement for their medical fees. Private-owned companies can always find an excuse to fire patients without violating the law. Stigma is a major reason for that; another pragmatic consideration that forces work units and companies to take work positions away from HIV/AIDS patients is related to the issues of health insurance and medical fees. Nearly all insurance companies in China refuse to provide health insurance to HIV/AIDS patients; therefore, medical expenses of HIV/AIDS patients become a potentially huge burden that none of the work units or companies is willing to carry. The "institutional affairs" Xiulan mentioned have much to do with this pragmatic consideration of the hospital. The hospital will never consider making an HIV/AIDS patient like Zhanshan an official staff member, or having any formal relation with him, though they count on him to help with many programs.

Zhanshan's expression of his feelings of grievance and unfairness reminded me of his radical self-criticism in his view of stigma associated with HIV/AIDS. Rather than being interpreted as embodiment of self-stigmatization, his self-criticism would be better understood as the way he tries to survive the enormous stigma associated with HIV/AIDS. In the face of stigma, Zhanshan and many other patients have no alternative but to accept what stigma has brought upon them. Stigma becomes a fundamental condition or premise that they have to accept and legitimatize in order to survive the extremely limited social spaces created by the broader social context to focus stigma against individuals with HIV/AIDS. That is to say, people who have HIV/AIDS have no choice but to accept whatever they are given while using self-criticism to adjust and alleviate their feelings of grievance and unfairness. They are remaking their emotional responses to stigma by using self-criticism against themselves to legitimatize stigma; they are remaking their moral experiences through remaking their emotional responses. Even though the emotional conflict might have been absent in public, it has never disappeared from the hearts of the stigmatized. The interior emotional conflict represents a gap and confrontation between two facts that people with HIV/AIDS have to face up to: owing to HIV/AIDS, they become non-persons and are no longer given what they deserve as normal persons, their work efforts and achievements have been ignored, unacknowledged, and underevaluated; on the other hand, in their interior world they remain normal persons who still have the same emotional feelings and value judgments normal persons have; they still have the feelings of grievance and unfairness when they perceive that they are treated as non-persons in their work and daily lives. Therefore, Zhanshan's self-criticism constitutes a critique rather than confirmation of the concept of self-stigmatization.

The Fourth People's Hospital's dining room was divided into two parts with two separate entrances: The infected area for all doctors and nurses on duty; the uninfected area for administrative staffs and other personnel, including staff working at the AIDS Care Center. Everyone used a rechargeable card to buy meals from the dining room. Nearly every day the AIDS Care Center had several visiting patients. In general, when it was lunchtime, Ding, Zhanshan, and I went to the dining room to buy meals for everyone and brought the food back to the Center, and then we had lunch together. Sometimes when more than 10 patients came in, we were short of hands and had to ask several patients to come with us, helping us buy food from dining room and bring it back to the Center.

One day when we were having lunch together, Ding told us that a few days before at a hospital's conference some staff from other clinics blamed the AIDS Care Center for bringing HIV/AIDS patients to the dining room and claimed it constituted a threat and danger to other staffs' health. Ding refuted this criticism and restated, as she had done many times before, that HIV/AIDS cannot be transmitted through daily contacts. In the end, the vice president of the hospital who was in charge of the AIDS Care Center stood up against this criticism by saying, "We are all medical professionals working at a hospital specially treating infectious diseases including HIV/AIDS. If we have this wrong opinion and attitude against HIV/AIDS patients, how can we educate other people in this society to change their minds and attitudes toward these patients?" This story once again confirms that stigma does exist even if people have the correct knowledge about HIV/AIDS and even within a hospital featuring treatment for HIV/AIDS. Stigma associated with HIV/AIDS has much to do with how people with HIV/AIDS are perceived in the local moral world rather than with how much people know about this disease.

To be honest, I have to admit that, during my first several days at the AIDS Care Center, I did not feel comfortable when I had lunch together with Zhanshan and other patients. Although I knew how HIV/AIDS is transmitted and that daily contacts, such as eating together, won't cause infection, I was still fearful that it is unsafe and dangerous. My fear had nothing to do with my knowledge condition of HIV/AIDS and its infection routes. As time went on, however, I got used to this feeling and learned how to control it; I felt more at ease when I had meals with Zhanshan and other patients. Sometimes when we were eating, Zhanshan and Xiulan said to me, "I didn't touch this part (of the dish), you can have it if you want." I had never refused their kind offers even I was almost full, but the fact was that during that period I always had a good appetite partly because I did a lot of volunteer work every day. Zhanshan and Xiulan often laughed at the way I ate. One day, they said to me, "Watching you eating makes people feel life is great."

Yang Ping

Yang Ping was in his first year of college when we met each other at the AIDS Care Center. He was also HIV positive. At the time, Yang Ping had not begun receiving HAART treatment because his CD4 count was still more than 200.[9] Once a week Yang Ping came to the Center to pick up a special soup made from Chinese herbal medicine, which was believed to be able to enhance HIV/AIDS patients' immune system and keep their CD4 counts above 200 in order to postpone the day they have to start taking anti-virus medications that have potential to cause significant side effects on patients' livers. On his first several visits to the Center, Yang Ping often burst into tears when someone tried to speak to him. Later when Yang Ping became familiar with us, a shy smile came to replace sadness over his face. But that smile had never made us feel better for him. Everybody feels sympathetic for Yang Ping at the first sight of him, a short and thin boy, always wearing a worn sweat-soaked T-shirt. It took him an hour and a half to ride his bike to get to the clinic from where he was living.

Yang Ping was born into a rural family in a village of Henan province, which had been known as one of the poorest provinces in China and recently had become a major site of the HIV/AIDS epidemic due to prevalent blood selling practices across the province over the late 1980s and early1990s. Yang Ping did not get AIDS directly from selling blood, but he was also a victim of it. Several years before when he was in high school, Yang Ping was infected through tainted blood transfusion at a local hospital, the blood he received was the product of blood selling.

---

[9]CD4 is a glycoprotein located on the surface of T-cells that control the human immune system. Therefore, CD4 count is indeed the number of the T-cells containing CD4. CD4 tests are important in assessing the human immune system and the efficacy of treatment in the case of HIV/AIDS. In general, HARRT treatment starts when CD4 count is less than 200. CD4 count implies which stage of the HIV life cycle patients are in. In my field experience, CD4 count became a major daily concern of HIV/AIDS patients, and for them the number "200" also carried a special meaning because it draws the distinction between HIV carriers (CD4 above 200) and AIDS patients (CD4 lower than 200). In the daily conversations among HIV/AIDS patients, CD4 count remains a main topic, in addition to viral load. They were so anxious about their own CD4 counts that they took frequent but unnecessary CD4 tests; however, the more tests they took, the more anxious they were.

When I asked Yang Ping about the blood selling in his village, he burst into laughs and seemed to have forgotten he was a victim. "It was called blood economy, which local governments had approved and advocated as a promising policy of developing the local economy. During that time, many local work units built their own stations for blood selling; even schools and local finance bureaus had their own blood stations. Nearly everyone in my village went to sell blood for money at the time. Everyday I saw lots of people heading to those blood stations to sell blood; they walked together like they were going to the city for shopping as they did on holiday days." The local hospital where Yang Ping received his blood transfusion also set up its own blood selling station, which was the biggest one in his county. Even those peasants from nearby villages also came to sell blood for money. "Every day was like a holiday," Yang Ping added. Thousands of people who had participated in this "blood selling campaign" were infected by HIV.[10] However, none noticed it until more and more people who sold blood in the past started to die mysteriously. By the year 2005, among the people who were infected through selling blood, only 200 were alive.

When Yang Ping was in high school, he accidentally fell to the ground and had a slight cerebral concussion. Yang Ping was immediately taken to a local hospital where a doctor strongly urged him to receive blood transfusion, which Yang Ping and his parents found out later was absolutely

---

[10]The population of Henan province is around 100,000,000. In the late 1980s and early 1990s, the officially registered blood stations were 80 while the illegal blood stations were countless. The number of people who were infected by HIV through selling blood in Henan has several versions. In 2004, the number officially released by Henan province was 11,000, while WHO estimated that it was around 100,000; in 2005, Henan province officially updated this number to 25,000 (sample was 280,000), but Dr. Zhang Ke from Beijing questioned this number and believed that the number is between 140,000 and 470,000. He conducted research in 10 blood stations in Henan and found out that each blood station has 50 beds on average, working 10 hours a day, 300 days a year while each blood seller sold blood 50 times a year on average. As he estimated, each blood station could have caused 3,000 people infected from 1994 to 1996. He also pointed out that the infection cases in Shangcai, a county of Henan province, should have exceeded 10,000. The fact is that the actual number remains unknown to date according to the information from the Chinese CDC.

unnecessary in the case.[11] It turned out that the blood Yang Ping received at the time was HIV positive. That is how Yang Ping was infected. But nobody knew it until 2003 when Yang Ping's mother heard that the county was providing a free HIV test at local CDC.[12] Since it was free, Yang Ping and his mother both had their blood samples drew and tested, and the test results indicated that the mother's sample was yin xing (negative) while the son's was yang xing (positive).

"At the time my mother and I did not even know what yin xing or yang xing means. The nurse who handed us the test results did not tell us either. When we two were guessing who was ill and who was not, a doctor came over and told us that I have HIV. Other than that, we heard nothing from those doctors; they did not tell us what to do or where to go for help". Yang Ping still had that shy smile on his face while speaking, he continued, "if there were no free HIV test in our county in 2003, I bet I would not know I am HIV positive even today."

Yang Ping described his tragic experience in a comedic manner. Soon he started to blame his mother rather than the local hospital for the deadly blood transfusion causing his HIV status. Yang Ping complained that his mother had never paid much attention to him; otherwise he would not

---

[11] During the reform toward market economy within the medical system in China, in the face of radically increasing competition in the market of medical services, many doctors often intentionally tended to over diagnose patients' diseases and give patients unnecessary and expensive diagnostic tests and medications in order to make extra money; on the other hand, they misuse some medications with patients in order to receive sales commissions and even bribes from the pharmaceutical companies who produce these medications. Owing to these prevalent medical misconducts, hospitals and medical staffs have been cast into a public image of greed and inhumanity: They care for nothing but money; while the professional morality of medical staffs has widely been called into question among the general population, which further increases the distrust between doctors and patients and results in more and more lawsuits concerning the incidents of malpractices within medical institutions. Owing to the increasing tension in doctor–patient relations, patients and their families often violently attack medical professionals out of anger whenever there is a unexpected result of treatment. Some vagrants even find a job out of this situation and are called yi nao (people who intentionally cause trouble to hospitals and medical professionals in order to get money); they would like to be hired temporarily by patients' families to attack medical professionals.

[12] CDC, Chinese Center for Disease Control and Prevention.

have been infected. "She just did not care much about my daily life, such as eating, schooling, and health. As any rural woman does, she basically cares less about these things because of lack of education. She simply has no idea about these things; on the other hand, she does not have much time to take care of these things after working in the fields for a whole day. What matters most to her is to make enough money to feed the whole family and pay my tuitions."

Yang Ping's criticism of his mother for her negligence reminded me of Zhanshan's self-criticism. They both expressed the feeling of helplessness. In the face of threat and danger caused by the insecure and chaotic broader social context, there is little a single person or family can do about it; rather, they have no choice but to accept the reality and try their best to protect themselves. If anything bad happened to them, they have none but themselves to blame; they tend to attribute their tragedies to their own carelessness in the face of threat and danger that are simply far beyond their control.

After Yang Ping tested HIV positive, his family gradually found out that they were not alone and the same tragedy fell on about 200 people in their village. Regarding themselves as innocent victims of the malpractice of the local hospital, Yang Ping, his family and all others who were in the similar situation went to the local hospital and then to the local government for explanation and justice. However, the local hospital and government both remained silent on this issue and shifted responsibilities onto each other. These victims eventually decided to send several patients and their families as local representatives, including Yang Ping and his parents, to Beijing to shang fang (appeal to the highest authorities for help and justice).[13] So they did, but it ended up with nothing after they had

[13] "Shang fang" originates in ancient time and has a long history in China. It refers to a practice that local people appeal to the higher authorities for help and justice, which they cannot seek from local authority because of corrupted local judiciary. It is not formal appeal in the sense of law but a personal moral practice of speaking out of personal grievance and asking for justice. In ancient time, local people either went to the capital to appeal to the highest authorities, including the Emperor or central justice department, or stepped in the way of imperial envoys patrolling across the country to speak out their grievances. In today's China, this tradition remains. When local people believe that corrupted local administration or justice department is involved in the injustice done to

stayed in Beijing for several months; instead, Yang Ping missed his entrance exam to college. After they came back to village from Beijing, Yang Ping attended another high school to prepare for the exam of the following year. For Yang Ping, life was still going on after all, though none seemed to be willing to take the responsibility for the apparent injustice done to him. He could not afford waiting any longer. At the new school, Yang Ping told his teacher the truth why he missed the exam in the year before, and then he was immediately kicked out of the classroom. After that, he had to transfer again, and this time he decided to conceal his HIV situation and told nobody about it.

In 2004, Yang Ping took the exam and received admission from a college located in Beijing. When the chair of the department in which Yang Ping was studying heard about his HIV status, he demanded Yang Ping to quit right away. Fortunately, a journalist whom Yang Ping used to know during the process of shang fang helped him persuade the chair to let Yang Ping stay; however, the condition was that Yang Ping was not allowed to live in the college's dormitories. Yang Ping had no choice but to move out of the dorm and rent a place off campus to live. As a compensation, the college waived Yang Ping's tuition.

The place Yang Ping rented for living was a basement, which the landlord was generally prohibited to rent out to people for living under the legal regulations in Beijing. It was not a place for people to live but a storage room without bathroom, kitchen or even windows; nonetheless, it was the only place that Yang Ping could find and he had to accept it. Every Thursday Yang Ping rode his bike an hour and a half to the AIDS Care Center to pick up free Chinese medicine soup. He spoke of how he had HIV as if he were telling a funny story and always had that permanent shy

---

them, they go to Beijing, the capital, to appeal to the central justice department for help and justice. In general, they have to stay in Beijing several weeks, even years, trying to find connections to higher authorities in order to speak out their grievances. Although governments at all levels set up special offices to receive people for shang fang and collect their appeals documents, people generally insist to speak to someone in charge in person about their grievances, which is unrealistic most of time. There are so many people going to Beijing for shang fang from time to time that the places they usually stay during the process of shang fang become fixed in some suburbs of Beijing and came to be known as "shang fang cun" (the villages for shang fang).

smile on his face; sometimes he could not even help laughing at his own narratives of what happened to him. But those moments always made people who were listening start to sob in their hearts.

Yang Ping's appeal to the local hospital, the government, and the judicial system, and even the highest central authorities for help and justice had been turned down in part because the local hospital and government were involved in the blood selling campaign that caused his infection. Although the sufferers are always likely to blame corrupted administrations and judicial systems when they fail in their appeal for justice, simply attributing the failure to corruption does not help us understand the whole situation created by HIV/AIDS epidemic. It is not just Yang Ping and the other patients who have similar experience and their families, but also the medical system, the administrative system, and the judicial systems that have to face up to the tragedy.

Yang Ping's failure in appeal for justice has to be relocated and understood in the broader political context in China. In general, the government at any level has more power than the judicial system at the same level. The government actualizes total control over the society through its dominant control of all available social resources. Behind the government at all levels is the hierarchical system of the Communist Party in which the Party Secretary has the ultimate right to make decisions on any issue. The social administration in China is mainly based on "red-headed" documents, such as official notices, orders, policies, and even leader's personal replies,[14] which are often stipulated without considering the established laws. They have the political power to go beyond and even replace the latter. Owing to its compromised independence, the judicial system in China in fact does not possess an independent authority outside the control of government. If the local judicial system wants to deal with injustices related to the local government, it has to appeal to the higher

[14] Red-headed document is an official document with its title and seal in red, is issued and passed downward within governments and other administrative institutions. The documents issued by different institutions often conflict with each other. For example, the documents within the health care institutions demand the local health care institutions to provide free condoms at hotel rooms for the sake of safe sex; while the documents issued by the institutions of public security identify the presence of condom as an important evidence of committing the crime of prostitution.

authorities for permission to practice the law. In the face of the cases like Yang Ping's, even if the government is dealing with a single case, the concern for societal stability often replaces the idea of personal justice. Owing to the increasing number of such cases in China since the late 1990s, the local judicial system received a notice from the higher authorities demanding them not to accept the cases of HIV infection caused by tainted blood transfusion.[15] The higher authorities were fearful that many hospitals run by the state involved in these cases would go bankrupt if they lost the lawsuits and had to pay the possibly huge sum of compensations; and on the other hand, if the judicial system accepted these cases, it would have developed into a collective social campaign against the local medical system and even the local government, which would probably lead, it was feared, to societal stability. The reason why Yang Ping and many other patients' appealing for justice had been turned down by the judicial system is the political economics of dealing with the epidemic of HIV/AIDS in China.

On February 17, 1993, the Ministry of Health of China issued a notice named Basic Standards for Blood Collecting Stations (*weiyifa*, No. 2, 93), which started to add blood tests to the procedures of collecting blood. Included were tests for HBsAg, HCV-Ab and HIV-Ab.[16] This notice implies that before that day in the practices of collecting blood there had been no such tests at all or such tests had not been taken as necessary or legally compulsory procedures. July 14, 1995, the Ministry of Health issued another notice (*weiyaozhengfa*, No. 55, 95) demanding that the blood products that have not been tested are not allowed to be produced and are prohibited in clinic use. The two notices indicate that the collection, production and clinic use of infected blood before the dates the notices were issued had not violated the orders of the Ministry of Health or the law at the time. Therefore, the blood stations, pharmaceutical companies and hospitals do not have to fulfill their

---

[15]This notice cannot be verified, but a lot of patients I met in field mentioned it and told me they heard so from local judicial system. I believe it was an informal notice circulated within judicial system.

[16]HBsAg is the surface antigen of the Hepatitis B Virus, indicating Hepatitis B infection. HCV-Ab refers to hepatitis C antibody; HIV-Ab means HIV antibody.

legal responsibilities for the possible infections they caused before that dates.

The two dates started to carry special and important meaning for people who are infected with hepatitis or HIV through tainted blood collection or transfusion if they decided to sue the blood stations, pharmaceutical companies or hospitals that they thought caused their infections. It really matters what time, even precisely on what day, they sold blood or received blood transfusion. Time issues become one of those factors that can determine if they have a chance to win the suit and get financial compensation. More importantly, these patients have to present evidence, such as the evidence related to hospitalization, blood transfusion, and the blood test results right before and after the incidence of selling blood or receiving blood transfusion, to the court of law in order to prove that they were infected through tainted blood collection or transfusion rather than other infection routes such as sexual intercourse or intravenous drug injection. Nonetheless, most of HIV/AIDS patients had not realized that they were infected until years after they were eventually diagnosed. They cannot present all the evidence needed. Therefore, in general it is very difficult for these patients to win a suit, if not impossible. For instance, Yang Ping told us about what happened in his own experiences of appealing for justice, "It (his blood transfusion) was a long time ago. At the time, we had no idea about this disease, how could we know we were supposed to keep those documents as records? That's ridiculous. In fact, I did not even take HIV test at all no matter before or after the blood transfusion because none knew about it at the time. The local hospital might keep the copies of those documents, but I am not sure. You know, those small hospitals might not be managed properly as you expect. Besides that, if I am going to sue the local hospital, I don't suppose they are going to give me the documents I need."

People infected with HIV through tainted blood collection and transfusion play a large part in the epidemic of HIV/AIDS in China, which is unique with respects to the epidemic in the global context in which the major HIV infection routes are sexual intercourse and intravenous drug injection. In the face of the epidemic of HIV/AIDS in China, patients and their families run into a critical life crisis that most of them cannot survive without the help from outside; on the other hand, the government have to balance two sides in dealing with an institutional crisis: Bringing justice to the victims and sufferers while protecting and helping the medical system survive the self-destructive consequence caused by its own misconduct. However, the government's management and its concern for social stability over personal justice have reinforced stigma associated with HIV/AIDS from the very beginning. It is in dealing with the threat and danger caused by the epidemic of HIV/AIDS to social stability that the government has helped create, maintain, and strengthen greater threat and danger to HIV/AIDS patients while producing and reinforcing the feeling of social insecurity and mistrust among the general population who are more likely to stigmatize HIV/AIDS patients. This is one of the major arguments I will further explore in the following cases.

For patients who are infected by tainted blood collection or transfusion, besides the difficulty in getting medical compensation, stigma constitutes an injustice for which they have nowhere to appeal for justice. Compared to HIV/AIDS patients who are infected through sexual intercourse or intravenous drug injection, people who are infected through tainted blood collection or transfusion are generally regarded as innocent victims, but the title of innocent victim has never protected these patients from stigma. The following two cases illustrate how these innocent victims are stigmatized in their local communities and even families.

Shufen

Shufen and her husband both had been working as teachers at a middle school in a county of Shanxi province for ten years. In 2000, Shufen made a blood donation through a volunteer activity organized by the school where she was working. Several days later, she received a phone call from the local CDC asking her and her husband as well as their two children to come in for blood tests. So they did. The test results turned out that Shufen and her 4-year-old daughter were both HIV positive. It happened so suddenly that Shufen felt faint and almost fell to the ground on the spot.

Back home the couple could not eat or sleep. "I almost broke down at the time," Shufen said, "my husband and I both know each other very well since we got married, and we have been wei ren zheng pai (moral persons). We have never been involved in any immoral sex. We are not that kind of person. We have never used drugs either. How could I get AIDS? I simply could not figure out why it happened to me."

Later the couple recalled a blood transfusion that Shufen had received several years before. In 1996, at a local hospital Shufen received a blood transfusion right before she gave birth to her daughter, her second child. It was that blood transfusion that Shufen and her husband believed caused her and her daughter's HIV infection.

"We felt fearful, hopeless and desperate. We were fearful that other people would know about our HIV situation. We began living our lives like thieves, always looking over our shoulders. Once other people found out our secret, my whole family would become wenshen (the evil of plague) in their eyes." After these years, Shufen still appeared shaken when she recalled those nightmarish days.

"But you cannot hide a secret forever. Our HIV situation was somehow exposed in 2001. Soon there was a rumor that spread across our small town, saying that all of my family members have AIDS. Wherever we go, there were always some people pointing at us from behind. If we run into someone, he or she will immediately shun us while covering mouth and nose with hand. When we go shopping, the bosses of stores became fearful and started waving to us as we got close, shouting at us, 'Don't touch my stuff, go away.' They did this to us the same way as they did to those homeless people. They waved us away like they were driving away flies. That was not the life a normal person deserves to live. My family became hongshui and mengshou (floods and brutal beasts, meaning great scourges) in other people's eyes. There was no way to live on. We just could not live anymore." Shufen burst into sobs and barely finished sentences.

Later she told me a sad story about what once happened to her older son, who is not HIV positive but who also has to suffer the family stigma. One day, her son came home and told her that his friends would not eat mo (a steamed daily food made of wheat in northern China) made by his family. "My son said that his friends were required by their parents not to eat our homemade mo because they were told that my son had a disease. My son asked me what kind of disease he has." Shufen said, "I felt I was stabbed in the heart. But I didn't feel it right to tell him the truth. So I just told him that he does not have any disease, and that his friends' parents said this because they wanted their children to be polite and not to eat other's food carelessly. I also told my son not to eat his friends' food as well. That was what I could do."

Shufen remarked that her family started bearing a new special identity in the local community after she and her daughter were diagnosed as HIV positive. The new identity often brought her family into an awkward situation when they were facing other families in daily life. In the past, when her co-workers, friends, and neighbors were hosting ceremonial occasions, such as weddings, funerals, and having babies, she always brought gift money (liqian) over to attend these family events and stayed for the banquet offered by the hosts, but after her family HIV situation was revealed in public, she often had difficulty in deciding whether she should go to these parties or not. "After I had AIDS, I just went over and gave my best wishes and gift money to the hosts, and then I would leave immediately. I would not stay or have meals with other guests."

"Did they ever invite you to attend these family events after you had AIDS?"

"No, they did not."

"Then why did you still go over there?"

"Let me tell you how I understand these things: if they don't invite me, that's their faults because they don't show me their respect; but if I know these events and I don't go over to express my best wishes, that's going to be my fault. That is the sense of being a moral person, as I understand. I cannot give up my sense of being a moral person just because they lost their sense of being moral persons."

"Did they ever ask you to stay for a meal?"

"Some people did, but I could tell that they did not meant it even when they said so. On my side, I didn't want to stay there because I felt ashamed and also I didn't want to put the hosts in that awkward situation. You know, they have to care about how the other guests feel about me. I understand that. I just felt that I no longer have the face of being a moral person (mei lian zuo ren), though I still try to be one."

Family ceremonial occasions, such as weddings, funerals, and having babies, are regarded as important family events in Chinese daily life. They provided the sites where local moral meanings, interpersonal relationships, and social networks are displayed, practiced and reinforced. The way the ceremonial hosts organize these events (sending invitations, presiding over events, and offering banquets) and the way the guests attend these events (offering gifts, attending the banquet) have much to do with the local moral sense of being a person who has the sense of renqing (literally human emotions, meaning being a moral person who knows how to make interpersonal relationships and social networks). Both sides have to act and react in the proper morally regulated way. Yan Yunxiang, in his *The Flow of Gifts*, presents a detailed description of how family ceremonial events and gift exchange are managed in a village of northern China in the late 1980s and early 1990s. In his book, Yan states, "A formal invitation is sent only to those important guests who are close relatives or best friends and who live outside the village community" (1996: 48); however, "It is not unusual for oral messages to replace written invitations for the sake of convenience. More importantly, within the village community there is no invitation issued, and the host merely announces the hosting of a ceremony in advance through informal channels of gossip and chatting" (1996: 48). Yan further points out that there are several reasons for "the absence of formal invitations to guests within village community". "First, villagers feel that there is no practical reason to send a written invitation to someone who resides just across the street or on the other side of the village. ... Indiscretions in the sending of invitations are regarded as irresponsible and greedy; namely, they attempt to force others to attend the ceremony in order to accumulate monetary gifts. To avoid such implications, villagers are always careful about sending invitations. ... Ideal gift giving should be based on the donor's intention to give, rather than on the social pressure created by invitations. This is actually the logic underlying why there is no need to issue invitations within the village community" (1996: 48–49).

Sufen's situation in the local community reminds me of what happened to Guiying, a mentally ill patient I write in chapter two, in the village after she was found psychotic. The thought that there is no need to issue formal invitation within the local community implies that it is a common sense for people to attend ceremonies hosted by other families in the local community. However, it is this common sense that conceals the fact that some people are not welcomed to attend these ceremonies. Yan notes how villagers refused to attend ceremonies to show their dissatisfaction toward the host families, which usually are considered dead doors because of their incapability and inflexibility in making guanxi. He also mentioned how social status plays its part when people have to decide whether or not to attend a ceremony. He cites a story, in which a "careless and muddleheaded" cook working in the town government hosted a wedding ceremony for his son. The cook invited many cadres in the local government to attend the ceremony, yet it turned out that "only a few cadres actually attended the wedding". For most of cadres, "they felt obligated to attend the wedding and offer gifts, according to the rules of gift exchange, but to be so close to an ordinary cook, and especially one who had a reputation for stupidity, was an embarrassment" (1996: 135–136). Yan's cases show how people refused to attend the ceremony hosted by dead doors and people with higher social status are not really obligated to attend ceremonies held by those with lower social rank. He also describes how people are refused to attend the ceremonies. "The four bad elements had serious difficulty in gift exchange during radical periods of socialism when class struggle was emphasized" (1996: 158).[17] "They are forced into a dilemma. On the one hand, they did not dare to offer gifts in public to villagers with good class labels or cadres because they might be accused of attempting to seduce the latter. On the other hand, they also worried that their failure to offer gifts might be interpreted as a denial of previous gift — giving relations or as a violation of renqing ethics" (1996: 158). Therefore, "they would deliver a message in advance, by some secret channel, to ask the host whether they should attend the ritual" (1996: 158), otherwise, their gifts would be publically rejected.

Both Shufen and Guiying were in the same dilemma as the four bad elements. Shufen and her family members all belong to the unwelcome group because of her family's HIV/AIDS situation. Shufen and her family used to receive invitations from these events before she contracted AIDS, but after that they were no longer invited to attend any ceremonial event. Their identities of being normal persons have no longer been acknowledged; they are excluded from the group of normal persons and

[17]The four bad elements: landlord, rich peasants, counterrevolutionary, and rotten element (Yan 1996).

have been ignored, shunned, and avoided by the local community. In other people's eyes, Shufen and her family have become ones who do not deserve to be invited or be treated as normal persons because they are not considered normal persons anymore. Stigma associated with HIV/AIDS is the reason that Shufen and her family no longer receive invitations after her AIDS status was found out in the local community. When it comes to the ceremonies held in the local community, stigma implies who is not supposed to be invited. The absence of some groups in these ceremonial events is invisible, it disguises the critical breakdown of interpersonal relationships and social networks that happens to those groups who do not fit the cozy and harmonious image featuring the daily practices of local moral senses; it hides social suffering caused by social exclusion from the public. In the Chinese context, stigma implies the breakdown of renqing and guanxi, and reveals the boundary of renqing and guanxi.

Although Shufen do not receive invitations anymore, she still gave her best wishes and offered gift money to the host but skipped the banquet. On the host's side, Shufen showed up as an unexpected guest; on Shufen's side, she was trying to maintain previous interpersonal relationships and social networks by continuing the practices of giving gift. Shufen was still trying to practice as a moral person does, though she was no longer one in other people's eyes. Yan Yunxiang also mentions the "unexpected guests" who shows up in ceremonial events, "At most ceremonial occasions, there are unexpected guests who take the initiative to show up and offer gifts; the more such guests like this, the greater the social face of the host" (1996: 49). Apparently, Shufen was not that kind of "unexpected guest" who is expected to bring social face to the host; instead, her presence in ceremonial events might cause the host to lose social face. Therefore, considering her absence in the banquet would do well to both the host and herself, Shufen offered her gift money and left the event quickly. Her absence meant that she understood the host's situation and cared about how the host and other guests felt. She, as a non-person to the host and other guests, cares and understands others just as a moral person is supposed to do. Shufen's decision of offering gift money but not attending the banquet indicated that she was aware of being a non-person in other's eyes, but she still tried to act as a normal person and maintain her dignity of being a moral person in her own perspective. Her responses to the situation inflicted by stigma show us how a stigmatized person tries to live a moral life.

HIV also ruined Shufen and her husband's teaching careers. After Shufen's colleagues found out her AIDS situation, they would no longer get close to her, or talk to her face to face. Even her office became a prohibited area; her co-workers who used to share the office with her began moving out one by one. Meanwhile, Shufen noticed that even her students also started shunning and avoiding her. Whenever she stepped into the classroom, her students immediately began covering their mouths with their hands. Shufen said, "I felt a pain in my heart when I saw my students doing this to me. The pride and dignity of being a teacher I used to have are all gone. But I had to stand it. I just could not imagine what it was going to be if I lost my job." Several months later Shufen realized that her last hope, keeping her job, was going to be taken away.

One day, a relative came to visit Shufen, asking,

"Do you have that disease?"

"I am just HIV positive, not an AIDS patient."

"Then you'd better leave, I mean, quit your job. The principle of your school asked you to do so. I am just a messenger. The principle told me that many students' parents submitted formal complaints to him and he does not have another choice."

A week later Shufen was forced to quit her job "on her own will". Soon her husband also quit for the same reason, though he is not HIV positive. Shufen's son was also forced to quit the kinder garden he was attending at the time, though he is a healthy child free of HIV too. The other families complained that they could not let their own children stay with a kid from an HIV family, and they even threatened the director of the kinder garden, saying that if Shufen's son stayed they were going to have their own children transferred to other schools. Under that pressure, the director had to ask Shufen to take her son home. Shufen tried to persuade the director and other parents to believe that her son is as healthy as other children; she even brought her son's blood test result signed by the local CDC to the kinder garden and showed it to the director. But all of her efforts failed. After that, her son had to stay at home all the time. None of other local kinder gardens would accept him; he also lost all of his friends, nobody would play with him anymore. In 2002 after the Chinese Spring Festival, Shufen could no longer stand that her son had to go through this painful situation, she made a decision and sent her 4-year-old son away to live with a family relative in another town.

Shufen burst into tears, "He was only 4 years old. I could not just watch his life getting ruined because of me." Since Shufen sent her son away, she has not paid a visit to him for a long time; she was fearful that her presence would ruin her relative's family. During that period what she could do was make phone call once a week to check on her son. Every time when she was on the phone with her son, they both began crying. "I cried at this end of the line, and my son cried at the other end. My son asked me why I sent him away and if it was because I didn't like him. He said he missed me and wanted to come home. That really broke my heart. I didn't know what to say, I just cried. After that, I don't dare to make that phone call anymore because I was afraid to hear his cries. It really tore my heart apart. So I just looked at his photos when I missed him, crying while holding his photos in my hands." It has been four years since Shufen sent her son away. During the four years, Shufen only visited her son six times. "I have no idea when this kind of life is going to end."

Shufen's efforts of maintaining her identity and dignity of being a moral person did not improve her family's situation of being stigmatized. Her whole family, including her husband and son who are HIV free, was stigmatized and excluded from the local community. Both Shufen and her husband were forced to quit their jobs, and their son was forced to quit school and was even sent away into a kind of exile. They were driven out of all public areas and kept from being seen in public. The social mechanism underlying stigmatization has changed from stigmatizers' shunning and avoiding the stigmatized to the stigmatized's shunning and avoiding stigmatizers; namely, stigmatizers' fear of the stigmatized is replaced by the stigmatized's fear of stigmatizers. The threat and danger meant by the public to the stigmatized replaces that meant by the stigmatized to the public.

Meimei

Meimei was 9 years old when I met her and her father, Zhiwei, at the AIDS Care Center in 2006. Seven years before, shortly after Meimei's mother, Ying, died of AIDS, Meimei was also diagnosed HIV positive at the STD Clinic of the Fourth People's Hospital in Beijing.

In 1997, after giving birth to Meimei at a local hospital in Hebei province, Ying was urged by doctors to receive a blood transfusion in order to recover sooner from giving birth. Ying and Zhiwei accepted the doctors' suggestion without hesitation, but things did turn out as the doctors promised. Rather than recovering soon from giving birth, Ying started having a strange disease with a symptom of persistent high fever. Half year later she could not even get out of bed. In 1999, Ying died without knowing what kind of disease she had. The same tragedy that had happened to Yang Ping fell upon Ying and her baby daughter.

For Zhiwei, it was the beginning of a nightmare. The fact that his family had two members who were infected with HIV aroused a panic among villagers. The neighbors who used to frequently visit this family began shunning and avoiding Zhiwei and his daughter. Meimei's friends would no longer play with her. Zhiwei had spent all of the money the family had saved in the past in order to get medical help for Meimei, but the thing he could not stand most was the way people in his village looked at Meimei and him.

I asked Zhiwei about how villagers had responded to his family HIV/AIDS situation. He started with a long sigh, "everything has changed since Meimei was diagnosed with HIV positive. I used to have a lot of friends in the village. They often came over to chat, play cards and drink. But after that, they all disappeared and never came back. They were frightened off. I could feel that even my family members, my brothers, sisters and even my father were fearful, though they did not say it to me. I could tell that they were also avoiding Meimei and me. Actually I too felt scared in the very beginning. My brothers and sisters had been living with us together for years, after that they all moved out for fear that they might contract HIV or be discriminated against. They told me that they did so for the sake of their own children's safety and asked me to understand their situation. I was really angry and could not forgive the way they treated Meimei and me. They asked me to understand their situation, but why couldn't they understand my situation and how I feel? I simply could not understand why my family members did this to us: gave up on us as those villagers did. But later when I calmed down, I came to understand how they felt at the time. They had their own concerns and had to protect their own children. You know, when kids play together, sometimes they hurt themselves or each other. That happens a lot. Parents cannot watch them 24 hours. What if Meimei got hurt and started bleeding? That could be dangerous to other kids within the family. I understand that. So now I understand why they moved out and left us behind. I don't blame them anymore. If I were them, I might have done the same thing."

Zhiwei thought back to the early days of his family tragedy. "In the beginning, I stayed at home all the day because I felt ashamed. I was afraid to leave home and look into other people's eyes. I was so fearful that I would not even leave home. Sometimes when I had to go out with Meimei, I could feel that everybody in the village was avoiding us. Meimei was three years old at the time. Nobody dared to touch her. Even when she fell to the ground, nobody would help her. That would have never happened to her if she were a healthy child. One day, Meimei asked for candy, I gave her 20 cents and she went out to buy candy. Several minutes later she came back happy with candy in her left hand and the 20 cents I gave her in her right hand. I asked her why. She told me that the old man who sold candy didn't want her money and gave her candy for free, and then urged her to leave quickly. She was happy with the free candy. She was too young to understand what was going on. But I knew why. The old man was afraid of her and didn't dare to take the money from her hand, which was why he didn't take the money. All of children in the village have been avoiding Meimei. Wherever she goes, other children immediately run away. Nobody wants to get close to her."

After Meimei was diagnosed HIV positive, Zhiwei initiated a lawsuit against the local hospital that gave the blood transfusion to Meimei's mother. Every time when Zhiwei went out for the lawsuit, he had to bring Meimei with him because he was the only one who would take care of her. "Sometimes I took Meimei to those shopping malls to have fun. I could not afford anything, thus we were just doing window-shopping. Meimei liked to play with the motorized stairs in shopping mall. She often took those motorized stairs up and down for fun. She was happy and satisfied with that. But when I looked at other children accompanied by their parents buying new clothes and fancy toys, I didn't feel comfortable; you will never know how I feel in my heart. I felt xin suan (a feeling of sourness or bitterness in one's heart). I cannot imagine that was the childhood I could give to Meimei, and that was the childhood she could get." Tears formed in Zhiwei's eyes.

Zhiwei's lawsuit against the local hospital ended up with nothing because he failed to present adequate evidences required by the court. He was so angry and desperate at the result that he once thought about revenge and suicide: Kill the head of the local hospital and then bring her daughter to Beijing and commit suicide in public at Tian'an Men Square in order to let his grievance go public. "But I cannot just let this family shame and suffering go like this," Zhiwei said, "I have to live on to clear our names even it is only for Meimei." In 2002, with the help of several lawyers from Beijing, Zhiwei's lawsuit and family tragedy went public. Many people across the country made donations to the poor family. In 2004, the local hospital was sentenced by the higher people's court in Hebei province to pay Zhiwei a compensation of 360,000 yuan. Zhiwei won the lawsuit but had never really received the compensation ever since. "Over these years of being in the lawsuit, I always felt that there was some unknown power intervening in the normal administrative and judicial processes. I heard that the head of the local hospital had many connections to some powerful figures. He had a lot of relatives who were working for the governments at the level of county, city and onto province. I was told by the court that they had no way to force the hospital to execute the court's final sentence: pay the compensation."

In the face of a similar situation, Yang Ping failed to make his case into a lawsuit against the local hospital; Shufen and her husband had no choice but to quit their jobs and send their son away to hide from the public; while Zhiwei won the lawsuit but still could not get the compensation. Being innocent victims did not protect them from being stigmatized in their local communities. Moreover, Zhiwei and his daughter experienced stigma within family. Zhiwei's brothers, sisters, and even father all moved away from the family and left Zhiwei and his daughter behind, rather than helping each other in the face of so greatly difficult a family situation.

During the Culture Revolution, as the political propaganda of "class struggle" spread across the country, traditional Chinese culture was criticized and delegitimatized, even family values were undermined, and family relationships were replaced by class relationships. Political campaigns introduced the idea of "class struggle" into families and pitted family members against each other; husband and wife, parents and children were urged to draw a distinction between each other and treat each other as "class enemies". Nearly 40 years later, under the social pressure created by stigma associated with HIV/AIDS, although Zhiwei's father, brothers, and sisters did not aggressively attacked Zhiwei and his daughter, they did draw a distinction between themselves and Zhiwei by moving out. By doing so, they not only moved away from the threat and danger posed by HIV/AIDS but also kept themselves from being stigmatized. In Zhiwei's view, his relatives forsook their family values and no longer treated Zhiwei and his daughter as family members. However, in the relatives' perspective, they moved away out of concern for their own children, and they forsook Zhiwei and his daughter in order to protect their own families. In this sense, Zhiwei's relatives might be accused of being immoral (forsaking Zhiwei and his daughter) by doing moral things (protecting their own families). To quote Arthur Kleinman, "So here we have a contest between radically different moral justifications" (2006: 21).

In his *What Really Matters*, Kleinman states, "Danger arises when our most deeply held values and emotions are threatened or lost. And people themselves become even more dangerous when they feel that these things are at serious risk" (2006: 18–19). "A real danger threatening the moral order… is associated directly with the other group or indirectly blamed on them. This leads to the second-order, and often more deadly, danger of the threatened group either actively or passively acquiescing to the destruction of the people perceived as the source of that threat" (2006: 19). In Zhiwei's case, his daughter's AIDS posed a threat and danger to his relatives; out of concern for their own families, his relatives moved away and stigmatized Zhiwei and his daughter. It was in protecting their own families that the relatives created a greater threat and danger to Zhiwei and his daughter. Zhiwei's blame of his relatives and his relatives' stigmatization of Zhiwei and his daughter are based on the same moral sense: protecting one's own family. In this sense, rather than being generally accused of an immoral and inhumane practice, stigmatization is also based on local moral sense and is applied as a must-do moral practice in daily life.

Yang Ping, Shufen, and Zhiwei all are innocent victims of HIV/AIDS epidemic, but they failed in appealing to authorities for justice. This occurred no matter how innocent they were and how hard they tried to seek help. Their failures have strengthened the feeling of social insecurity and mistrust that all people experience in their daily life. Under increasing social pressure created by the radical social transformation ongoing in today's China, none feels his/her life is secure; social mistrust has accumulated due to people's growing feeling of social insecurity. People began to suspect everything, including the government, hospitals, the judicial system, other people, and even their own relatives. Yang Ping, Shufen, and Zhiwei trusted hospitals. They also trusted the judicial system, but the latter turned them down and had never brought them the justice they expected. Trust turned their lives into a nightmare. Living in a society featuring social insecurity and mistrust, not knowing where the potential danger is located and when it will attack, and expecting neither help nor justice from any institution, people have no alternative but to avoid potential dangers and protect themselves. They can count on no one else for protection. To quote a typical reply from people I interviewed, "Those people [people infected with HIV through blood selling or blood transfusion] are miserable and pitiful. I do feel pity for them. But what if I got hurt or infected if I stay with them? Then who is going to help me? Who is going to speak for me? Who is going to take responsibility for that? Nobody!" This statement expressed a strong feeling of social insecurity and mistrust; nonetheless, it provides us an angle to look into the social logic underlying stigmatization. Social insecurity creates social mistrust; while social mistrust, in turn, strengthens social insecurity. Social insecurity and mistrust mutually constitute each other. In a broad social context featuring social insecurity and mistrust, people tend to stigmatize others associated with threat and danger in order to protect themselves. Therefore, they create a greater threat and danger to the stigmatized. They participate in stigmatization in order to overcome the threat and danger posed by the stigmatized. Stigmatization is embodied in denying and disapproving people's personhood in the local moral sense, reducing them into non-persons, cutting off their interpersonal relationships, breaking down their social networks, excluding them from public areas, compromising their social spaces, and limiting their life chances.

Even innocent victims among HIV/AIDS patients are stigmatized, not to mention those who contacted HIV through sexual intercourse or intravenous drug injection, which are viewed as evildoers of moral responsibility. The following cases are devoted to HIV/AIDS patients who are widely believed to deserve the punishment embodied both in the disease and in the social exclusion it creates.

Fangfang

Fangfang was one of patients who frequently visited the AIDS Care Center. She was originally from Hunan, a province in southern China. Ten years before when she was going to marry a workmate, both of them tested HIV positive.

In 2006, Fangfang was working for a company from which she certainly had hid her AIDS situation. At the time, her CD4 count reached 9, the lowest I have ever seen among the patients visiting the AIDS Care Center. In her situation, she should have started anti-virus treatment much earlier; however, she had been worried about the side effect of the treatment and did not want to start taking medications. Especially when she observed what the treatment did to Xiulan, whose body fat had been displaced and accumulated onto her back after she had been taking anti-virus medications for years. Body fat displacement, one of the side effects resulting from HAART, generally occurs to women patients and makes their back look abnormally thick. The side effects of HAART not only do harm to patients' physical and mental functions but also disfigures patients by changing their bodies.[18] Fearing possible disfigurement, Fangfang was quite hesitant about whether to start treatment, though doctors strongly urged her to do so immediately.

During my research period in Beijing, another AIDS care program was organizing a painting workshop on weekends. Every patient was paid

[18] Side effects of HAART include: dizziness, nausea, insomnia, headache, diarrhea, liver failure, numbness, mental confusion, nightmare, dry skin and body fat disappearance or displacement.

60 yuan each time for attending this workshop. I went to the workshop several times with some patient friends I made at AIDS Care Center. Fangfang was one of them. One Saturday when I was sitting next to Fangfang on a double-decker bus headed to the workshop, I had a talk with her. It was early in the morning; except for Fangfang, several other patients, and I, no other passengers were on that bus; we were sitting on the second deck far from the driver. The following is the story Fangfang shared with me then.

In 1996, Fangfang and her husband took a blood test right before they were going to marry each other. Her husband was from Thailand and they got to know each other during work. However, what happened after several days would make the plot for a dramatic movie. "I still remember that day," Fangfang said, "early in the morning, my home was suddenly surrounded by several ambulances, and then several medical staff, all wearing white uniforms and masks, rushed in and escorted everybody they found in my apartment, including my parents and brothers, to get in the ambulances, and then drove us to the local CDC where it was demanded that we take the HIV test. It turned out that my husband and I were both HIV positive." After ten years when Fangfang recalled what happened to her family that day, she was still fearful. She kept repeating some details, such as the presence of several ambulances, white uniforms, and masks. She was also angry at the way her family had been treated by the medical personnel, "You cannot imagine how brutal they were! They treated us as we were some dangerous and disgusting beasts."

Fangfang turned away to look out the bus window, and then started sobbing with her back toward me, saying, "It is a shame. What I cannot stand most is that even my parents and brothers have to bear this shame and be humiliated this way."

After that, the local government urged Fangfang's husband, a foreigner with HIV, to leave China and go back to his own country, Thailand. "At the time, I felt so ashamed myself. I did not have the face to stay in my hometown any longer, so I decided to leave for Thailand with my husband." Fangfang seemed to have mixed emotions toward her hometown: fear, disappointment, anger, and hate. She said, "That place was so inhuman to us. I hate those people forever. They do not have any sympathy or conscience; even my family's relatives looked at me in a strange way at the time. They don't have any sense of renqing." Fangfang stopped and then added, "I will never go back to my hometown in my life."

Regarding the following years of living in Thailand, Fangfang described it as a fuzzy dream she hardly remembered. "I had been acting like an idiot; my head was all messed up. I did not dare to leave home, did not remember when to take a bath or change clothes, and did not know what to do or what to think. Actually, I cannot even remember what I had been going through over those years." According to Fangfang's narrative, she and her husband had been receiving HAART treatment in Thailand; for the treatment result, however, she said, "it seemed those medications did not work well on me."

In 2005, Fangfang heard that a hospital located in Beijing began applying traditional Chinese Medicine to HIV/AIDS patients. She wanted to give it a try since she had always been worried about the side effects caused by western medications and she believed that Chinese medicine is free of side effects. That was why she came back to China. However, her husband's visa was rejected and he was refused entry into China because he is a foreign AIDS patient. Therefore, Fangfang had to travel to Beijing alone. The time I met her at the AIDS Care Center, she already had started taking the special Chinese medicinal soup, but her AIDS situation became critical and her health condition worsened.

Ding and Zhanshan tried to persuade Fangfang to start anti-viral treatment, but Fangfang was still afraid of the possible disfiguring effect and had been hesitant about when to start treatment. She said, "I am still young; I don't want to look like that. That is horrible. So ugly." In addition, Fangfang had another issue, money, to worry about. She found a job in Beijing to make a living. With her salary, she could barely afford to live in Beijing, including rent and daily expenses. If she decided to receive treatment in Beijing, she had to pay for medications by herself, which she could not afford. That is related to a policy issued by Chinese central government in 2003.

Then the State Council issued a policy named "four free and one care" aimed at the spreading epidemic of HIV/AIDS (State Council, No. 7, 2004). The policy states, hospitals are to provide free anti-viral treatment for HIV/AIDS patients who are rural residents or urban residents who do not have health insurance; the CDC and health institutions at all level are to provide free volunteer consulting and testing for HIV; hospitals assigned to treat HIV/AIDS patients will provide free medication to prevent mother-baby transmission of HIV/AIDS and free HIV tests to babies; local governments will provide free education for HIV/AIDS orphans. In addition to these four free services, the governments at all level will provide financial support and subsidies to HIV/AIDS patients and their families who have difficult family financial situations, and help HIV/AIDS patients who are capable to support their own lives and improve their living conditions through self-help.

In the initial phase of this program, free medications were only supplied to AIDS patients who contracted HIV through tainted blood transfusion. Having been questioned about why it is not available for other HIV/AIDS patients, the Ministry of Health claimed that they were just testing the program in its initial phase, and after the pilot phase this program was to be expanded to cover other AIDS patients. No matter what the real intention was behind this test phase of the program, its practice again strengthened the impression among the general population that patients who are infected through tainted blood collection and blood transfusion are innocent so that they deserve free medication; while the rest of HIV/AIDS patients, such as intravenous drug users, sex workers and gay men, are responsible for their own diseases and do not deserve free medication. In this sense, this policy has, to some extent, reinforced the stigma associated with HIV/AIDS.

At the time I conducted research in Beijing, all AIDS patients were receiving free medication no matter how they contracted HIV; however, there was another issue that could and did prevent patients from accessing free medications. According to the rules issued within the health care system, free medication is to be administered and distributed in terms of patients' hukou (residency permit or household registration).[19] For example, if a patient has residency permit in Beijing, he/she has to

[19] Hukou, a system of residency permit or household registration, identifying a person as a resident of an area and recording relevant information, such as the person's name, birth date, nationality, marriage status, and other personal information related to other family members including parents, brothers and sisters. Hukou system started in China in the 1950s and has been used to prevent rural residents from moving to urban areas in order to protect social stability.

go to the Beijing CDC to get registered as a local patient, and then he/she can pick up free medications from the Beijing CDC; if the patient leaves Beijing but keeps a residency permit for Beijing, he/she is not able to access free medications from places outside Beijing; or if a patient who has residency permit of another province comes to Beijing without changing that residency permit, he/she cannot get free medications from Beijing either. However, the reality is that this residency permit based policy cannot keep up with the radical social mobility created by the floating population, which refers to about 130 million migrant workers who are traveling between rural and urban areas, and between different urban areas in today's China. Although residency permit plays a less important role in many areas of Chinese daily life than it did in the past, it carries special significance for HIV/AIDS patients when they try to access free medication.

In addition, owing to the stigma associated with HIV/AIDS, a lot of patients, if they can afford it, generally go to places far away from their hometowns to take tests, seek counseling, and receive treatment. They are fearful that their HIV/AIDS situation would be revealed in their hometowns once they have themselves registered at the local CDC; In that case, as a patient said to me, he cannot live anymore if everyone around knows he contracted HIV. Therefore, many patients would rather waive their right to free medications and buy medications by themselves from other places. Part of my daily volunteer work at the AIDS Care Center was helping Ding mail out medications requested by patients living outside of Beijing. Some of them were originally from Beijing and have residency permits for Beijing, they left for other places to make a living after they found out that they had contracted HIV; however, most of the patients who requested mail service were living in other provinces where their hukou were registered. They had been buying medications from Beijing since they started treatment. In general, patients living outside of Beijing sent their money to the AIDS Care Center and placed the money as a deposit under the management of Ding. When they run out of medications, they will make phone calls to Ding, asking for more medications, and then we buy the medications from the clinic, pack and mail them out at the address patients previously provided. Ding once reminded me not to put the address of the AIDS Care Center on the mail package because of patients' request. They are fearful that mailmen or other people could figure out their HIV/AIDS situation if they saw "AIDS" on the package.

In Fangfang's case, she is originally from Hunan; thus she has her residency permit registered in her hometown in Hunan. Therefore, she has no access to the free medications provided by the Beijing CDC. But she can get free medication from her hometown if she goes back to her hometown to get registered at local CDC; however, that is the last thing Fangfang would do since she has a great hatred of that place. Although free medications are offered to all HIV/AIDS patients, the hukou system makes free medications unavailable in reality to many patients. The hukou system has further limited HIV/AIDS patients' social spaces and reduced their life chances, which were already suppressed and limited by stigma associated with HIV/AIDS. I once talked to an official who was with the Chinese Center for Disease Control and Prevention, he agreed with me that the barrier created by the hukou system already prevented patients from accessing free medications; he also said that the CDC already noticed this problem, but the hukou system is administered by Public Security institutions under the control of the Ministry of Public Security; thus the CDC can do nothing about it. In China, the call for reform of the hukou system has been heard since the 1990s. Although the control of the hukou system has been weakened since then, there is no sign yet that this system will come to an end soon.

Haitian

Haitian was another patient friend I made at the AIDS Care Center. He presided over some activities organized by the Center, such as a learning English club, a health education program aimed at gay men's group. At the time I was helping him with these activities.

Haitian was tall, pale, and skinny, about the age of Zhanshan. He had been a government employee for almost thirty years. Twenty years before he married a woman, though he knew he always liked men rather than women. "At the time, Chinese had no idea about what gay is; we, gay men, didn't know of it either. As many people like me, I thought I was kind of abnormal and felt ashamed for it. Anyway, I got married as many of us did at the time." Haitian said, thinking back to the 1970s.

In fact, Chinese literature citing homosexuality dates back to ancient times; homosexuality has a long history in China.[20] But after the Chinese Communist Party took over the country in 1949, homosexuality was deemed a sexual crime till 1997 and remained a mental disorder till 2001. In today's China, although homosexuality is no longer regarded as a category of mental illness or a crime, and the society also seems more and more tolerant of it, homosexuality, in fact, goes underground; it has been absent, intentionally ignored, in public discourses. Gay men have never been paid public attention until the epidemic of HIV/AIDS began shedding light on this group. In China, homosexuality starts to draw public attention because it constitutes a major infection route of HIV/AIDS, while preventing HIV/AIDS becomes the major way to talk about homosexuality in public discourse. Official acknowledgment of the existence of homosexuality does not lead to social acceptance of it. Strong stigma is associated with homosexuality in Chinese society. As a matter of fact, in Chinese daily life, homosexuality has been considered something abnormal and immoral; it not only arouses disgust and disdain among general population but also poses a serious challenge and threat to family values, and also creates frustration and despair within families who have gay family members. The frustration and despair caused by having a gay man within the family is very much similar to the ones resulting from having a mentally ill person at home. Many gay men decide to hide the truth from their families because they feel ashamed; moreover, they are fearful that their parents could not endure the truth. They deem telling truth, revealing their homosexual identity, to their parents as "unfilial" behavior that is going to break their parents' hearts and make them blame in how they have raised their children. Two decades before, Zhanshan and Haitian hid their homosexual identity and married women because they did not recognize their homosexual identity at the time; while among the young generation of gay men in today's China, under the social pressure and family

---

[20] Chinese scholars believe that the earliest citation of homosexuality in Chinese literature can be found in *Shang shu-yi xun* compiled in Shang dynasty. The author warns people to keep away from being obsessed with beautiful boys. In fact, most documents are found to have recorded the homosexual relationships between ancient emperors and their love partners. See *Zhongguo tongxinglian yanjiu*, Liu Dexinn,

pressure caused by stigma associated with homosexuality, most of them still tend to hide the truth from their families and marry women, though they are now aware of their homosexual identity.

In 1999, Haitian found out that he contracted HIV when he went to a hospital to take a blood test, part of the routine health tests offered by his work unit. He went to the test together with one of his workmates. That was how his work unit found out that he had AIDS. Later his work unit informed him that his work position will be kept and he will get his wage as well as other benefits, but he does not have to go to work anymore. That way Haitian "retired" soon after he was diagnosed with HIV positive. Haitian commented on how his work unit responded to his AIDS status, "They [work units] always do so in that situation. They told me that they did so for my own good, and also for other workmates. They said, 'that way you don't have to come to your office and feel uncomfortable in front of your workmates, and your workmates won't panic either. Otherwise, there is no way to keep the work running. So it is good for all of us.' To be honest, I also thought it is a good solution for both my work unit and me."

Given the position Haitian held at his work unit before he retired, he would have had a promising career future. But now everything is gone. Haitian often expressed his regret when we happened to touch this topic during our conversation. In the beginning, Haitian always hesitated to talk about his family. Later when we became more familiar with each other, he started talking. Shortly after he was diagnosed HIV positive, Haitian told his wife that he was gay and had already contracted AIDS. "That was like a bolt from the blue. She was shocked, frustrated, and angry because I had been hiding my gay identity from her over those years, and then she got panic about my AIDS status. I suggested that we'd better get divorced. But later she refused my suggestion. She was afraid to tell her parents about everything, considering her parents' age and unstable health condition. In fact, I told none within my own family. I didn't tell my own parents either. My wife was fearful that everyone, including her parents, friends, and workmates, would find out I had AIDS if we got divorced. That is going to be a big shame. So we didn't go for divorce but decided to live apart. However, my wife was fearful that our parents and friends would found out what's happening if we live in separate places. So we just pretend to live together and hide my AIDS status from everyone else. In fact, we are still living together in the same apartment as we had been before. My wife bought herself a new set of furniture and utensils, including cookware, dining utensils, storage furniture, washing machine and bathroom furniture. Basically, we are still living in the same apartment; but we are not sharing anything. Even the space we are using at home and the period of time we are spending at home came to be marked and classified. We both remind ourselves not to go beyond the boundary. There are some spaces I will never go and some things I will never touch. We are avoiding seeing each other at home and always trying to leave when the other is coming home. In general, I am staying at home during day time while my wife is away for work; in the evening before the time she is about to come back home from work, I will go out, leaving the whole apartment for her, and then I will come back late at night. Only when our parents or friends come to visit us, we have to stay together and pretend to be husband and wife."

"How long have you two been doing this at home?" I asked.

"Since the day I told her that I contracted AIDS. It was 6 years ago." Haitian replied, shrugging while making a dry smile. "I already got used to it," he added.

There were no statistics showing how many couples infected by HIV/AIDS divorced as Zhanshan and his wife did and how many of them still kept together as Haitian and his wife did. I heard from Ding that it is about a fifty-fifty from what she had observed at the AIDS Care Center. Ding said, "I always ask our patients to bring their spouses in so we can tell them what HIV/AIDS is, how to prevent it, and make sure that they know daily contacts do not transmit HIV/AIDS and they can still live together. I am just so sad to see that many couples break up for this disease. You know, family support is very important for our patients to fight this disease. There is no way they can succeed on their own without family support. But many spouses do not want to come in for counseling. For them it is a shame and loss of face." The strong stigma associated with HIV/AIDS not only prevents people from getting to know about HIV/AIDS but also creates distinction between husband and wife within families, if they do not legally break up.

Because of the fear of stigma, Zhanshan's wife left him in order to get away from the stigma, protect herself from HIV/AIDS, and get on with her own life; owing to the same fear of stigma, Haitian's wife refused to get divorced in order to hide the shameful family situation from other family members and friends. Observed from outside, stigma might appear more prominent in Zhanshan's case; however, it is in Haitian's case that the distinction created by stigma within the family reveals what stigma means, how stigmatization came into being within the family, and how stigmatizer and the stigmatized both try to live a moral life in the face of a critical family situation. The distinction within the family formed when Haitian and his wife, for fear of the threat and danger caused by HIV/AIDS, began classifying and dividing furniture, utensils, and even family space and time into pieces: some belonging to Haitian while the rest belong to his wife; they keep the boundary every moment in their daily lives, using separate space and time. Distinction, embodied in boundary, separation, and exclusion, is what stigma is mainly about. As distinction forms and reinforces through repetitive daily practices, stigmatization comes into being. In the face of stigma associated with HIV/AIDS, Haitian's wife decided to hide his AIDS status and keep the suffering to themselves out of concern for their parents and the fear that she and other family members might also contract the stigma. To hide the truth is to protect themselves and other family members from the threat and danger caused by HIV/AIDS. She hid stigma but she was practicing stigmatization herself against Haitian within the family. On Haitian's side, he had to accept being stigmatized by his wife in order neither to bring stigma to other family members nor himself to be stigmatized by other people.

Concealing HIV/AIDS status, ranging from removing the tag on medication bottles to hiding AIDS status from everyone else,[21] is a

[21] Part of my daily volunteer work at AIDS Care Center was helping patients remove the tag on medication bottles. In generally, patients came to the clinic and picked up their medications, and then they repacked the medications, removing the original boxes and the tag on the bottles of medications, throwing away all medication instructions. Some of them replaced the original bottles with used gum bottles they brought with them. They did all of this to prevent their medication from being revealed to the public. Nearly every patient who has a job chooses to put medications inside gum bottles, which is a good disguise,

common management strategy among all HIV/AIDS patients I met at the AIDS Care Center. In general, they hide the disease from people outside the family; within the family most patients tend to hide it from family members other than spouses; a few of them even hide it from their spouses. They conceal their disease for fear that their AIDS status might be revealed to the public and they would then be stigmatized. They hide also out of their concern for their family members, especially their parents. They often put it this way, "I am afraid to tell my parents about this. How can I tell them that I am a gay and now I have AIDS? I believe that this is going to give them a heart attack and they simply cannot stand this attack. Moreover, I don't want to see they are going to be humiliated this way at their age."

The following case is a dramatic story about concealment. Even though it might be read as a comedy, it is a sad story.

Xiaobao and Huimin

Xiaobao, a handsome young man from southern China, and Huimin, a beautiful native girl of Beijing were both in their twenties and contracted AIDS. Xiaobao had been hiding both his gay identity and AIDS status from his family because of stigma associated with homosexuality and HIV/AIDS, while Huimin's parents were the only ones who knew about her disease. Huimin's parents worried that sooner or later Huimin was going to leave them by themselves because of her AIDS, thus they would like Huimin to have a healthy baby so that they could have the baby's company even when Huimin passed away in the future. Although Huimin didn't think it is a good idea to have a baby, given her health condition and her parents' age, she did understand why her parents were so desperate for a grandchild.

Huimin eventually decided to help her parents realize their wish; however, as an AIDS patient, Huimin knew that she could hardly find someone to marry her; moreover, Huimin didn't dare to have her own baby by

---

thus they can take medications at ease even when they are at work. But nothing is risk-free. A patient once told me that he had a problem when one of his workmates asked him for a piece of gum after the workmate saw his gum bottles.

applying the procedure of preventing mother-to-child transmission of HIV. Under such circumstance, Huimin and her parents chose to adopt a child. According to the relevant policy issued by the authorities, anyone who is qualified for adopting a child must be married. Thus, the only choice that Huimin had was to find someone among her patient friends who was willing to marry her or simply feign marriage to her so she can get the certification needed for adoption.

Huimin asked around among her patient friends and tried to find someone available. It turned out that a feigned marriage was the only way to go, and so Xiaobao was targeted. At first Xiaobao refused this offer since he always kept to his gay identity. Yet later, under the pressure from many patient friends, he decided to help Huimin. Thus, Xiaobao and Huimin got registered as husband and wife, but they agreed that they were not going to live together. It seemed to be a win–win deal: Huimin was finally able to adopt a child to make her parents happy, while Xiaobao would not have to take any responsibility of being a husband and father, and he can still feel free to get on with his gay life.

The plan worked out smoothly in the beginning. The only problem was that they had to pretend to be husband and wife in front of Xiaobao's parents from whom Xiaobao hid everything except for the marriage. Fortunately, Xiaobao's parents were living in a small town far away from Beijing. Thus Xiaobao and Huimin did not have much to worry about. The baby adopted by Huimin is a very cute boy. Every time Huimin brought the baby to the AIDS Care Center, we were all attracted and everybody liked to play him. I noticed the baby seemed different from those Chinese babies I had ever seen: the baby has brown hair and blue eyes. Although I suspected that it is not a Chinese baby, I didn't feel it right to ask Huimin about it at the time. Later I heard from Zhanshan that I was right and the baby is a white boy abandoned by unknown people at a local hospital. Zhanshan seemed worried more about this issue than Huimin, he said, "This is going to be big trouble. What are they going to do in the future? What are they going to tell others about the baby? Now the baby is very young; it is hard to tell if it is a Chinese baby or a white baby unless you watch closely. But as he grows up, he will look absolutely different from Chinese. Look at his hair and eyes! Huimin and Xiaobao are both Chinese, how are they going to explain that they gave birth to a white boy?"

Zhanshan's worry did make sense because Huimin and her parents hid the adoption from all of their relatives and friends, whom were told that Huimin gave birth to this baby. Huimin and her parents were fearful that their relatives and friends would ask around why Huimin adopted a baby rather than having her own baby if they told the truth. And if so, they would have had to tell another lie to cover the first one. One lie leads to another. The more lies they tell, the more suspectable they become, and in the end Huimin's AIDS status would be revealed to the public.

But that was not the only issue that Huimin had to worry about; things became far more complicated than were expected. In the beginning, Xiaobao and Huimin both agreed that what Xiaobao needed to do for this feigned marriage was only to present himself at the registry office where they were supposed to have their marriage officially approved. However, as Huimin came to know what it really means to be a mother and what it takes to take care of a baby, she began expecting more from Xiaobao. Although Huimin's parents loved to help Huimin take care of the baby, she sensed something was missing: a real father is needed for raising the baby; more importantly, a father's presence helps the mental development of the baby.

One day, Huimin came to the Center, asking around about Xiaobao. We had barely seen Xiaobao because he didn't visit the Center often. From what we heard from Huimin, it seemed that Xiaobao didn't visit his own "home" or check on his "son" often either. In front of Zhanshan and me, Huimin started to complain, without awareness of the agreement she had with Xiaobao, "He [Xiaobao] barely showed up. I have not seen him for several months. I am not asking him to come to see me or help me on anything, but at least he should come over to see the baby. You know, baby definitely needs to see his father."

"Did you ever call him?" Zhanshan asked.

"I did. But he always said he was busy. He is busy all the time. But after all he is my baby's father, at least in the sense of law. He should pay several visits to the baby. That's all I want from him. I am not asking for anything else."

Huimin did not feel well that time; she had an inflammation of lymph nodes on her neck. Doctors suggested she have surgery immediately. But Huimin was working hard to make money while taking care of her baby; she hesitated about when to have the surgery. Her neck was so badly swollen that she could not even move her head. Sitting on a sofa and staring at nothing, she said, "I really *fan si le* (literally vexed to death)."[22]

At the moment, Zhanshan and I did not know what to say to comfort Huimin. After Huimin left, Zhanshan called Xiaobao, asking how his son is doing without mentioning Huimin's complaint, and then suggested Xiaobao make some time to check on his son. Xiaobao hesitated for a moment and then promised to pay a visit to his son soon. After one week Huimin showed up at the Center in high spirits. She said, "You know what? Xiaobao came to see his son last week. He even brought us some fruits and cookies." We were smiling at Huimin; she was so happy. Zhanshan laughed at her, "Now you are happy! I really envy you two."

After a few days Huimin had a surgery on her neck. Even though the surgery was painful and after that she had to come to the clinic to have the bandage changed every two days, she was really in high spirits those days.

However, problems always follow one another. From the very beginning, Huimin and Xiaobao hid the baby from Xiaobao's parents. Now Xiaobao's parents started asking when they were going to have a baby. Huimin and Xiaobao felt that they could no longer conceal the fact that they already had a baby, so Xiaobao had to tell his parents that Huimin already gave birth to a baby. Xiaobao's parents became extremely angry when they heard the news because they as grandparents were not informed when their daughter-in-law got pregnant and when she gave birth to the baby. On the phone they blamed the son for not telling them this important family event in advance and insisted to come to Beijing immediately to visit and check on their grandson.

Xiaobao and Huimin were facing big trouble. They didn't have a real "home", a place where husband and wife are supposed to live together, at all in Beijing since it was only a feigned marriage. They were not living together. Huimin was living in her parents' apartment with the baby, while Xiaobao was living in a separate place with his partner. But in a few days

[22] Fan, a Chinese daily expression of mixed feelings of being tired, irritated, vexed, frustrated, lost and confused. A common word used when people feel that they are trapped under troubling circumstance. They don't know what to do, where to go, or who to ask for help.

Xiaobao's parents were coming to visit and stay at the place that had never existed. What to do? Huimin and Xiaobao soon figured out a solution. They borrowed an apartment from one of their patient friends, and then they moved in and set up everything: bringing all kinds of stuff from their own places respectively to the new place to pretend that they were living together. So they were ready to receive and treat Xiaobao's parents. Xiaobao's parents arrived on time and the show was on.

After two weeks, when Huimin showed up again at the Center, she looked exhausted. We asked her how the show did go, and she burst into laughs, "What a mess! You can tell that. But it was fun." Huimin went on to describe how they pretended to be husband and wife, how they could not find anything at the new place, and how they almost gave the game away. During Xiaobao's parents' stay, Huimin and Xiaobao pretended to act like they were an intimate couple. To play the game as real life, they talked to each other in the way a couple is supposed to do, always starting with dear and honey; they had to share the same bedroom at night, though one slept in bed while the other slept on the sofa; they prepared meals together, though they could not find utensils or sauce at any time; they played the roles of father and mother for taking care of the baby, though Xiaobao always messed up with baby's diapers. In front of Xiaobao's parents they were trying to play the roles of husband and wife; when they were alone, they made jokes to each other on hit or miss. At the end of the first week of his parents' visit, Xiaobao could not stand it anymore, he was fearful that he and Huimin would give the game away sooner or later since there was no sign that his parents were going to leave soon. Thus Xiaobao suggested Huimin find an excuse for herself to leave home. Huimin had to do as Xiaobao suggested. She told Xiaobao's parents that she was going to be out of town on business for a while, and then she left.

This is all I know about Xiaobao and Huimin's story. I didn't have a chance to follow the further development of the plot. It seems that the story needs an ending. But, is there an ending to such a life full of concealment? Can concealment have a real ending? Is a feigned marriage all that Huimin asked for? For HIV/AIDS patients, concealment is everything; everything is about concealment. The tragic sense of Xiaobao and Huimin's story lies in the fact that in public, by concealing themselves and performing a moral drama, they can live a moral life in the sense that they can be socially identified and acknowledged; while in private, the moral sense embodied in their real life experiences of fighting the disease and stigma, defending their dignity, and protecting their loved ones might not be known or acknowledged at all.

Summary

In this chapter, I included cases representing several subgroups of HIV/AIDS patients, such as gay men (Zhanshan, Haitian, and Xiaobao), people who contracted HIV/AIDS through blood transfusion (Yang Ping, Shufen, Meimei, and her mother), and people who contracted AIDS from their spouse or boyfriend (Fangfang and Huimin).

These cases show that HIV/AIDS are stigmatized in medical system, school, justice system, local community, and family. Zhanshan complains that his work at the AIDS care center has never been officially recognized and appreciated because he is an AIDS patient; Shufen, Meimei' father and Yang Ping all appeal to justice system for justice but failed; Yang Ping is forced to quit school in high school and later to move out of college dormitory and live separately; Shufen and Meimei are both isolated and discriminated against in the local community; Fangfang and her family was first mistreated by the local CDC and then forced to leave the country; Haitian has to live a separate life at home to protect him and his wife from the shame; Xiaobao and Huimin have to pretend to marry each other in order to conceal their AIDS status.

Compared to people with mental illness, especially psychosis, HIV/AIDS status is relatively easy to hide from the public. Most of these patients have to live a double life: In front of people, mainly their family members, who know their HIV/AIDS status, they live as non-persons in the family but they have no family acceptance or recognition; at other times, they pretend to live as normal persons in public. A major concern for these patients is hiding their HIV/AIDS status. Many patients have to quit job, move to other cities, or simply stay at home doing nothing for fear that their HIV/AIDS status might be publicly exposed. They retreat from public sphere by cutting off relationships and quit social networks. Thus, they make themselves into non-person in society.

Chapter Four

Ethnography of stigma associated with HIV/AIDS in Yunnan

Dexin, Yunnan Province

Approaching the end of my research in Beijing, Dr. Meng, the director of the STD Clinic of the Sixth People's Hospital in Beijing, offered me a position in a HIV/AIDS project on which his clinic was cooperating with a local hospital in Dexin city of Yunnan Province. For me, it was totally unexpected, but I have to admit that it was exactly what I needed and had been looking for at the time. Dexin, the capital of Dexin Bai Autonomous Prefecture of Yunnan Province in Southwest China, is well known for a high level of ethnic diversity. Among the 56 ethnic groups in China, 26 are found in Yunnan. In the traditional or orthodox sense of anthropology, Dexin's exoticism makes itself an "ideal" site for ethnography. Moreover, Yunnan is said to be one of those provinces that has suffered most from drug use and HIV/AIDS; most of HIV/AIDS patients in Yunnan were infected through sharing needles in intravenous injection of drugs. The HIV/AIDS epidemic in Yunnan seems to be a quite different case from what happens to Beijing, at least from what I observed in the clinic where I conducted my fieldwork. Fieldwork on drug users, another important subgroup among HIV/AIDS patients, would help me to get to know and understand more of the epidemic. Therefore, I accepted this offer without any hesitation. Dr. Meng insisted that I should pay the site a visit before I make a final commitment. Although I already made up my mind that

I was going to do it no matter what, I did pay the site a one-week visit as Dr. Meng suggested. In the middle of December 2006, I took a flight from Beijing in the morning, and two and a half hours later I arrived in Kunming, the capital of Yunnan Province.

Yunnan is located in the most southwestern part of China, the province borders Guangxi and Guizhou Provinces in the east, Sichuan Province in the north, and Tibet Autonomous Region in the northwest. It shares a border with Burma in the west, Laos in the south, and Vietnam in the southeast. Yunnan province has a population of 44 million. It has been one of China's relatively undeveloped provinces. In 1994, about 7 million people lived below the poverty line of less than an annual average income of 300 yuan per capita. With an input of 3.15 billion yuan in 2002, the absolutely poor rural population in the province has been reduced from 4.05 million in 2000 to 2.86 million (*Kunming ribao*, September 11, 2007). Yunnan's major industries are tobacco and mining. The main agricultural products include fruits, flowers, and vegetables.

Owing to its unique landscapes (Yungui Plateau in the north; a limestone plateau with karst scenery, underground rivers, and deep mountain gorges in the east; various rugged mountains and rivers in the west), mild climate (Kunming, the capital of Yunnan Province, is known as "spring city"), and various ethnic minorities, Yunnan Province is one of China's major tourist destinations. Visitors include domestic and foreign tourists. The local government has been boasting the concept of ecotourism because of Yunnan's relatively low level of pollution than the rest of China. In 2004, tourism revenues amounted to 36.9 billion yuan, accounting for 12.6% of the provincial GDP (*Yunnan ribao*, February 10, 2006).

Dexin sits in the west of Yunnan, about 330 kilometers west of Kunming. Dexin city consists of an old town and a new town: the old is north of the new one. When I arrived in Kunming at noon that day, I decided to take a bus rather than airplane to get to Dexin. Dexin has its own airport, which is not common for such a small scale of city in China but indicates that Dexin plays a significant part in the provincial tourism industry. Dexin and Kunming are only a 40 min flight apart, but it took me 4 hours of bus ride on the highway from Kunming to the new town of Dexin. I then took a cab, and 40 min later I arrived in the old town, my destination, around 8:00 that night. I was welcomed by two workmates: Matt and

Vivian, who had been working on the project for a long time, and then they brought me to a dinner with Dr. Wang, the head of the Dermatology Clinic of Dexin People's Hospital, along with several other members from a local MSM education center that Dr. Wang supervised. They were all working on the project at the time. The project was conducted at Dr. Wang's clinic. In most of the general hospitals in China, HIV/AIDS patients receive treatment and care in dermatology clinics, because dermatology clinics have historically been the principle site for the treatment of sexually transmitted diseases like syphilis, gonorrhea and now AIDS.

After the dinner, I arranged to settle down at a family hotel owned by the parents-in-law of a nurse who was working at Dr. Wang's clinic. Hotels run by families can be found around the old town because of the flourishing tourism industry. Accordingly, a popular profession for many local people, more men than women, is driving cars or buses for tourists, which is called paoche (literally running cars) in the local dialect, a private business. The husband of the nurse I just mentioned was doing paoche business, and so was her father-in-law; her mother-in-law was managing the family hotel. According to the local government's statistical bureau, Dexin's tourism made 3.3 billion yuan in 2004, which is a quarter of its GDP (Dexin tourism monthly report, December 2004).

In contrast to the modern new town, the old one has an ancient look: it is surrounded by city walls on its four sides and on each side there is a gate. The local government was said to have decided to keep its old and new towns separate in order to create a time tunnel for tourists. The old town was originally built during the Ming Dynasty in emperor Hongwu's reign (1368–1698) but definitely had been rebuilt recently. However, behind the ancient look lies a different story. As a tourist destinations, Dexin is popular not only for its historic sites but also for the "Foreigners' Street" that features western-style bars and stores serving western style food and music. Some of bars and stores are owned by foreign business men from all over the world.

In its history, Dexin has been an important transportation hub, which has connected the southwestern border areas, even southeastern Asian countries like Burma and India, to the inland of China since B.C. 110–105. At that time, the Han Dynasty set up four counties in the Dexin area and placed them under its own control. In the 730s, under the support provided by the Tang Dynasty, one of the local tribes united the other tribes and established the Nanzhao Kingdom. In 902, the Nanzhao Kingdom ended in a palace coup and was replaced by the Dachanghe Kingdom; in the 920s, owing to continuous palace coups, the Dexin area was first taken over by the Datianxing Kingdom and then by the Dayining Kingdom. In 937 (Houjin Dynasty), a Dexin Kingdom was established through the military intervention carried out by a governor assigned by the central government and 37 neighboring tribes. In 1253, the Dexin Kingdom was terminated by the Yuan Dynasty's military invasion and the area it used to control was renamed Yunnan Province, a name it has kept since then.

The Dexin area originally was inhibited by a variety of ethnic minorities, of which Bai and Yi are the two biggest groups. According to the 2000 census, Dexin Bai Autonomous Prefecture had nearly 3.30 million inhabitants, among which the Han population was 1.66 million (50.35%), Bai 1.08 million (32.8%), Yi around 426 thousand (12.94%), and Hui 66 thousand (2.0%).

The local products in Dexin include marble, batik, carved woodworks, puer tea, mixian (literally rice threads, rice noodles), erkuai (a local pastry made of rice mixed with milk), rushan (literally milk fans, a local fried milk product), and plum wine. Dexin is so well known for producing marble that the city is named after marble, which literally translates as "Dexin Stone" in Chinese.

In the local dialect, Dexin generally refers to the old town, which is surrounded by the Cangshan Mountains to the west, Erhai Lake to the east, Shangguan to the north and Xiaguan (the new town) to the south. The local people often use the word fenghuaxueyue to characterize Dexin's geography and culture: Xiaguan's feng (wind), Shangguan's (in the north of the old town) hua (flowers), Cangshan's xue (snow) and Erhai's yue (moon). Fenghuaxueyue in Chinese is usually cited as a common euphuism to describe an idyllic life style full of gaiety, grace, elegance and decency, which in the native view is a perfect symbol to convey the romance and beauty of Dexin. Dexin has long impressed Chinese people with a poetic sentiment, to which a famous Chinese movie, Five Golden Flowers produced in 1959, has contributed. It is a romantic story about how five beautiful Bai girls find their handsome Mr. Right; the story takes place around a fountain called "butterfly spring" in Dexin. In the movie, the main actress is named Jinhua, golden flowers, and the main actor, her lover, is named Apeng, literally eagle. When the movie became popular across the country, people started calling all Bai girls Jinhua and boys Apeng.

However, the HIV/AIDS epidemic in Yunnan presents us with a painful image hidden under the surface of fenghuaxueyue. Yunnan has been the province that has the most HIV/AIDS patients in China. In 1989, 146 heroin users were reported being HIV positive in Ruili, a border city in Dehong Dai and Jingpo Autonomous Prefecture of Yunnan province. According to the official report released by Chinese CDC in 2007, the 146 HIV/AIDS cases found in Ruili in 1989 were believed to be the origin of the indigenous HIV/AIDS cases in China. By September 2003, 13,948 HIV cases, 841 AIDS cases and 526 death caused by AIDS had been reported in Yunnan. As of the end of 2005, HIV/AIDS cases had been diagnosed in 127 of 129 counties in Yunnan; among its 16 prefectures three were defined as in high transmission phase, 11 in mild transmission phase and two in low transmission phase. By 2006, 20 thousand HIV/AIDS cases had been found in Dehong prefecture, the infected cases represented 2% of the prefecture's population. HIV/AIDS was found among farmers, workers, cadres, police officers and school teachers. According to the data released from the Health Department in Yunnan Province, by September 2007, HIV cases mounted to 56,054 and AIDS cases were up to 5,036, death caused by AIDS was 2,211, while medical experts estimated that the province has at least 80,000 infected people.

Most of HIV/AIDS patients in Yunnan are intravenous drug users who have contracted the disease by sharing needles. Yunnan neighbors the notorious Golden Triangle, one of the most extensive drug-producing areas of Asia and of the world since the 1950s. The area overlaps the mountains of four countries of Southeast Asia: Burma, Laos, Vietnam and Thailand. Having been used as a major passage for drug trafficking, Yunna suffered much from the drugs flowing in from neighboring Vietnam, Laos and Burma. According to Yunnan Public Security Department, during the period from January to November in 2000, Yunnan Province cracked 7,630 drug cases, confiscated 765.6 kg of opium, 541.4 kg of "ice" (a common nickname for methamphetamine), and 2,881.5 kg of heroin. More than 4,300 suspected drug dealers were arrested. In 2005, China seized 6.9 tons of heroin and 5.5 tons of "ice", of which 4 tons of drugs were found in Yunnan. In 2006, Yunnan frontier police cracked 3,793 drug trafficking cases, arrested 3,764 suspects, and seized a total of 3,078 kg of drugs, including 1,429 kg of heroin, 763 kg of "ice" and 866 kg of opium.

Dexin People's Hospital is located next to the north gate of the old town. It has four major buildings. Compared with other hospitals in China, where outpatient and inpatient services are generally placed in separate buildings, Dexin People's Hospital instead arranges its space in terms of different clinics; for each clinic, its inpatient area and outpatient area are generally located right next to each other. The Dermatology Clinic, the Traditional Chinese Medicine Clinic, and the Gastrointestinal Clinic and Proctology Clinic occupied the same building, which has a typical Bai style[1]: a two-floor building constitutes the compound, which have a screen wall on the south, more than 20 houses on the other three sides and the main gate facing the east. The screen wall is decorated in snow white color, elaborate black ink drawing and Chinese characters. All the houses face inward. In the middle of the compound's yard there is a man-made fountain. A small scale rockery display sits in a pool where several colorful fish are raised.

The Dermatology Clinic occupies the west side of the compound and three additional rooms on the north side: one room on the first floor and two more on the second. On the first floor of the west side there are three rooms: A workshop where the doctors and nurses apply their special prescriptions to make ointment for skin diseases, a laboratory and Dr. Wang's office; on the second floor are an injection room with three beds, two diagnose rooms (one for HIV/AIDS and the other for skin diseases) and a nurse's station. On the north side, the clinic has a VCT (Voluntary Counseling and Testing) room for HIV/AIDS patients on the first floor and two more rooms on the second floor used as wards.

---

[1] Bai style architecture is called sanfangyizhaobi in the local dialect, literally three houses and one screen wall, meaning compound with three houses on each side and a screen wall facing the north where the main house sits.

The first HIV/AIDS case in Dexin was diagnosed in 1990. According to the information released by Dexin's local CDC, 1,222 HIV/AIDS cases were found in Dexin Bai Autonomous Prefecture in 2004. 77% patients contracted HIV/AIDS through sharing needles in intravenous injection of drug; 18% through sexual intercourse; 1% through mother-child transmission; 3% remained unknown. Among HIV/AIDS patients 45% are farmers and 37% are unemployed. (Huang *et al.* 2006) By the time I arrived at the end of 2006, Dexin People's Hospital's Dermatology Clinic had treated 118 HIV/AIDS cases, of which 105 patients were receiving treatment or health care at the time, six patients had already died, four patients had lost the contact with the clinic, and three other patients had quit treatment. During the period I was working there, the clinic had ten staff, including 4 doctors and 6 nurses, and 12 beds in total. In addition to his work at the clinic, Dr. Wang was also directing a women's health center (a health education center aimed at female sex workers) and a MSM education center.

In 1997, Dr. Wang diagnosed the first HIV/AIDS cases in this clinic; from that time on, Dr. Wang has been focusing on HIV/AIDS cases in addition to his patients with skin diseases. Dr. Wang recalled his early experience of working on HIV/AIDS. "At that time, the hospital didn't want to set up an HIV/AIDS clinic for fear that it would scare other patients away. So my clinic was set aside by the hospital to deliver basic health care to HIV/AIDS patients in private. We went to patients' homes to take care of them and we didn't even wear our white uniforms because patients and their families were afraid of disclosure of their HIV/AIDS condition. In fact, what we could give to patients at the time was very limited because neither medication nor real treatment was available. So we just tried to work on their symptoms in hope that they could feel better. Basically, what we could provide was to help those patients die decently. Most of time we were just doing terminal care. Many families left their members who contracted HIV/AIDS alone and didn't take care of them anymore; they felt it is not only danger but also shame that those patients brought to their families. Hence, a lot of patients were left alone and had to live an isolated life where nobody really cared for them. When we went to visit these patients, we actually offered them their only chance to communicate with other human beings. A patient once told me that I was the only one who would shake hands with him after he was diagnosed as HIV positive. His family just simply cut him off."

Based on almost 10 years of working on HIV/AIDS, Dr. Wang had made his clinic a model site for HIV/AIDS prevention and treatment in Southwest China. His clinic had been cooperating with many international foundations and health care institutes on HIV/AIDS. During my stay, the program on medication adherence I was going to join was ongoing at the clinic along with several other programs funded by Britain institutions, including a MSM and HIV/AIDS education and prevention program funded by Barry & Martin's Trust, and Peggy Health Center supported by Mary Kinross Charitable Trust.

Since early in the 21st century, under the pressure imposed by increasing international communication and especially the lightning like development of the internet, the Chinese government realized that they were unable any longer to deny or conceal epidemics or refuse international help in the way they did before. They had to take at least a slightly more open stance toward international and foreign help. More and more international and foreign institutions and funds became increasingly involved in dealing with the HIV/AIDS epidemic in China. Speaking of international technological and financial help, Dr. Wang expressed his appreciation but his worry as well, which is common among the Chinese medical professionals I have met. The worry is that all of this help is implemented in the form of long or short-term projects, but none knows for sure how long these projects are going to last. This makes long term planning difficult, if not impossible. Another issue is particularly related to the international or foreign funds coming with these projects. In general, patients get money for participating in these projects, taking HIV tests, or even attending lectures. Although the monetary promotion provided by international or foreign institutions did help patients actively get involved in HIV/AIDS prevention and treatment, it had never been applied by Chinese health care institutions in dealing with epidemics before international associations came into the country. The Chinese medical professionals are worried that the monetary promotion is going to "spoil" patients. Mrs. Ding in Beijing and Dr. Wang both expressed their worries about the monetary promotion: "this is going to make our own work much more difficult after these projects end. When there is no project, there will be no money". They strongly suspect that patients will still come back for education and training programs, HIV testing, or even take medication on time once these projects end. They believe that it might not be such a good idea to use money to buy patients involvement in education and treatment. In fact, the monetary promotion had already been misused according to what I observed at the AIDS Care Center in Beijing. The center was running a program aimed to help more gay men get HIV test. The information was distributed by several volunteers working for the center. Each person who comes in for test receive 50 yuan for compensation, while those volunteers also get payment depending on how many people they persuade to take the test. Subsequently, it turned out that many men who are not gay but pretending they are came to the clinic to take the test in order to receive money. Some volunteers even give information cards to people who they know are not gay men in order to get more money. Although it is good to have more and more people take HIV testing, the practices of this program violated its original design and damaged the credibility of the research results.

The Chinese government's attitude toward international associations is both ambiguous and contradictory, but it has its own worry, which is different from the one expressed by medical professionals. Governments at all levels welcome international associations in order to get the technology and funding needed to deal with the HIV/AIDS epidemic; moreover, by accepting this help, the central government shows to the international society that it wants to be part of the latter rather than to be seen as a stubborn and inhumanly tyrannical regime. This is a lesson that the Chinese government has been learning from increasing international criticism over its previous misconduct in disguising and concealing natural or social disasters, controlling information, and refusing international associations. However, the Chinese government also worries that its authority and control over its own population is going to be challenged owing to the influence of increasing international aids. The active involvement of international and foreign institutions in China may give Chinese sufferers the impression that it is the international and foreign institutions rather than the Chinese government that really cares about them and willingly helps them deal with their suffering; more important is that international and foreign institutions provide an alternative resource other than the Chinese government, which used to be the only resource provider in China. All of these challenges are perceived by the Chinese government as danger and threat to its own authority. In Beijing, Zhanshan told me that he had been warned and threatened by a district CDC officer to quit the AIDS Care Center he was working with and then join an official program under this officer's control. Zhanshan was warned that all HIV/AIDS patients should "tingdangdehua" (listen to the Communist Party) and "gendangzou" (follow the Communist Party) rather than other organizations; otherwise, there will be no hope for these patients. Although the AIDS Care Center is not a real NGO and this officer might be just another rude Communist cadre who speaks nothing but stale official parlance, the warning message delivered to Zhanshan and other HIV/AIDS patients did reveal that the Chinese government, out of the perceived danger and threat posed to its authority by the active involvement of international and foreign institutions in dealing with the HIV/AIDS epidemic in China, started competing with any other independent institution for patients.

In Dexin, the program that Dr. Meng introduced me into was aimed to monitor AIDS patients' medication adherence and examine the correlation between medication adherence and treatment effect. HIV/AIDS experts believe that medication adherence, taking medication on time, has a profound influence on treatment effect for HIV/AIDS. Poor adherence not only leads to less effective treatment results, but also causes early emergence of medication resistance, which means a specific combination of various anti-virus medications prescribed for a specific patient is no longer effective for this patient. In that case, doctors have to give the patient another prescription, if there is one. However, the reality in China that both doctors and patients have to face is that the free medications provided by the government are limited. Therefore, if medication resistance occurs to patients, doctors might run out of prescription options because no alternative free medication is available, which means there will be no medication for those patients who cannot afford other medications by themselves. In this sense, helping patients improve their medication adherence is to make a prescription effective as long as possible and postpone the day that medication resistant occurs. This is why the medication adherence issue is especially addressed in China, though it has been addressed everywhere in the world.

The medication adherence program operated at Dr. Wang's clinic was conducted by an American university that provided all the equipment and funding. The funding was managed by a third-party, a survey company located in Beijing. Dr. Meng in Beijing was hired as a Chinese advisor to this program. Before I arrived in Dexin, the program had been running for a year at Dr. Wang's clinic; by the time I arrived two field staff members remained in the program: One was an American student from the university which conducted this program, the other, whom I was going to replace, was a Chinese girl hired in China by the program. The medication adherence program was basically applying electronic medication bottles to AIDS patients on anti-virus medications. Once the electronic medication bottle is activated, it starts memorizing exactly when the user opens it to take medication. The bottle has to be refilled with medication every month. When patients come to the clinic for refill, the bottle will be placed onto a scanner, which reads the bottle's memory chip and outputs the medication adherence record: a dot chart, each dot signifies a time point showing when this patient opens this bottle of medication. Patients have their CD4 counts and viral loads tested every three months. The test results are analyzed together with patients' medication adherence records. At the beginning of the program, 88 patients in total were entered; by the time I arrived, 76 remained, several patients died of drug overdose, some moved to other cities, and the rest were held at a local detox center because they were caught using illicit drugs.

Dawei — You Make the Work Unit Feel Shamed

Dawei was one of patients I first got to know at Dr. Wang's clinic. In his early 30s, Dawei was short, pale and disabled. He was the most humble patient I met at the clinic. He barely talked except on the occasions that he had to answer questions from doctors and nurses. When he was going to leave the clinic after he had his medication bottle refilled, he always said "thank you" or "sorry for bothering you" to everyone with a humble smile on his face.

The second time I met Dawei, I asked him if I could interview him. He immediately agreed as if he was taking an order without any hesitation. This happens a lot especially when one is doing research in rural areas in China, where people usually do not have any sense that they have the right to decide whether or not to be interviewed. I often feel uncomfortable with this reality. It seems to me that I am forcing them to accept my interview request on account of cultural expectation, social power, and the simple decency of people. Although I do not use any word to coerce my informants, there is no doubt that my background, including who I am, where I am from, and what I am doing, definitely constructs a power-relative situation and that makes it difficult for potential informants to say no to my request. In this sense, any ethnographical encounter happening in field work is much more complicated than one simply modeled as researchers and informants. In my encounter with Dawei, my education background, my position in the project and my relationship with the clinic, and Dawei's being a drug user, an AIDS patient and a research subject in this project who had been taking over 150 yuan from my hands each month all placed him in a vulnerable situation where he could hardly say no to my request. In daily life, Chinese people usually feel it impolite to say no straight out to others, but in this situation, it has much more to do with the power-structured encounter rather than just trying to be nice.

As I always do, I told Dawei that he did not have to do it if he did not feel like talking with me. But Dawei replied immediately, "No, no, I have no problem with that. I would love to." This time it turned out that I felt I could not say no to Dawei. I had to comfort myself with the thought that talking to him is what he needed and might help him anyway, though he might not realize it — a way of justifying the interview which left me uneasy.

Dawei's disability was not caused by infantile paralysis as I assumed; instead, it was caused by an accident. He was born in a workers' family; his father and mother were both workers at local factories. When Dawei was five years old, he was playing at his father's steel factory and some equipment collapsed over him and left him crippled. This accident might not make any sense to people living outside of China. Why are parents bringing their children to the place where they are working? But it was very common in China in the past, particularly before the 1990s, when kindergarden service was not available. Parents had to work the whole day, and if no grandparents were available to help take care of children, parents sometimes had to bring their children to where they were working so they could do their jobs as well as take care of their children at the same time. Sometimes parents were busy and left their children unattended. This is how the accident happened.

We had our first conversation in a quiet room located in a separate building, where I was assigned to conduct interviews. Dawei attributed his social failure to the disability caused by the accident. "It is all about fate. This is my destiny." A regretful expression came to Dawei's face when he recalled the accident that caused his disability. He felt that his chance of being a normal person had been cut off ever since, "because you are disabled, you just cannot have a normal life as other people do. Your future is simply gone, and you have to live a completely different life."

After junior high school, Dawei did not continue his schooling. It was 1994 and he was 15 years old. Dawei's school experience seemed not that successful and he would not talk much about it. I asked him how he was doing at school and why he did not continue his schooling. He turned away and looked out the window, a bitter smile forming in his face, "I was not doing well at school. So I decided to quit. There was no need to waste time and money." I went on to ask him how he was doing with his classmates at school. Dawei glanced at me and looked down at the table between us, "you must know that," apparently he understood what I was trying to ask, "How a crippled kid will be treated at school? Nobody wants to be your friend, or even get close to you. They tease you all the time and speak out about your disability in front of you just for fun. They mock the way you walk in public in order to make fun."

I do remember something similar happened back in my elementary school days. After many years I realized that none other than the disabled children themselves has the strongest feeling of what the stigma associated with disability is like. I recalled that there was a boy, Jun, at my elementary school, who had a big but not that scary burn scar covering half of his face. None wanted to share a desk with him unless it was forced by our teacher. Jun was usually called by a nickname: his last name plus "bazi" (literally scarred face) when our teacher was absent. Fortunately, Jun's family was relatively rich at the time; he often brought some money to school so he could buy candies, comic books and other stuff to share with students who were sitting around him. He was trying to make some friends, but it had never worked well enough to improve his situation of being teased. It turned out that other students still kept calling him bazi and making fun of him after they enjoyed his generous gifts. Everyone enjoyed teasing Jun and wanted to see how he became angry and frustrated; none had ever paid any attention to how he felt about it. One day, I went to talk to Jun on a mission assigned by our teacher. I cannot recall what the conversation was about, but I still remember that he used "you people" to refer to me and the other students. I was shocked. In fact, at the time I didn't understand exactly what he meant by "you people". But it was the first time that I realized that the world in his eyes is somehow different from the one in my view. Years later I came to sense the meaning of "you people", it referred to the students who were liked by teachers, quick at learning and always followed teacher's instructions. Then who were "we people" to whom Jun believed that he belonged? It had to be the students who were slow at learning, could not finish homework on time and those who had disabilities such as stuttering, facial disfigurement, and motion weakness as paralysis. I also realized why we people, the "you people" in Jun's eyes, had never used "you people" to refer to Jun's kind of students, it was probably because they had never had a place in our view of the world. To some extent, they had never existed in our world because the way they exist did not matter to us. In Jun's eyes, the world is divided into two categories: you people and we people; while in our view, there is only "we" in the world, others are neglected, omitted and excluded because their existence does not matter in the world we people articulate. Nor need it matter from the standpoint of status, power and normality. We were the normal, the rest were outsiders or worse. If we try to reframe the concept of stigma in this context, it will help us understand how stigmatizers and the stigmatized perceive the world and how they see each other respectively. It also will further help us explore what the logic behind stigmatization is actually about.

For some students, school is a place where they can make progress and achieve something meaningful; while for others, school creates nothing but nightmares. Here is another example. I once met a college student during my field work. He quit college and then was hospitalized at a mental hospital back in his hometown. The reason was that he was seriously depressed because of what for him was an unbearable problem of smelly feet, which made him an object of hate in his college dormitory. In Chinese colleges or universities, several, sometimes even dozens of students have to share a bedroom. Under such a stressful living condition, the limited living space and the absence of privacy results in grievance, hatred, fighting, even murders. Many stories of this kind have been neglected, omitted, and excluded from the socially conceived beautified images of college and university life.

Dawei would not talk much about his school experience, but I could imagine what it was like from my own experience. He had been isolated, neglected, discriminated and stigmatized because of his disability. The stigma associated with his disability forced him off the normal life track. He chose to protect himself from being stigmatized by quitting school. Being stigmatized destroyed Dawei's identification with the dominant social ideology and community, but it had not broken his sense of belonging. After Dawei quit school, his parents tried to find him a job, but they could hardly find one because of his disability. "Even a normal person could have difficulty in finding a job, not to mention a disabled person like me," Dawei said. Most of the time, Dawei stayed at home and had nothing to do. Gradually, Dawei found some friends who were his schoolmates but who also had quit school. "They were like me. We were not that kind of school person and not good at learning. I think we just do not fit in school. So they made the same decision as I did. They did not have jobs either. Sometimes we hung out together, but basically we had nothing to do. Day by day nothing had really changed. You know what kind of feeling that is? You just feel that there is nothing in your life. Your life is blank. Nothing, absolutely nothing! You wish you could do something to make a day, but there was nothing really going on. Then every day you just wish that something would come up, even a little change would work. You hope that there could be something, whatever it is, that you can deal with."

Then something really came up. "One day, a friend showed up with this stuff, you know, drugs. That was how I started using drugs." Dawei glanced at me with a sorry smile on his face.

"Did you have any idea what it is at the time?" I asked.

"Yes, of course. We all knew about it."

"Then did you know that it could cause addiction and you could never get away with it?"

"Everybody heard about it. But we just did not really think that much. Also I believed that I could control myself. If I wanted to quit, I could do it anytime."

Later in my conversations with those HIV/AIDS patients who were infected through sharing needles, I heard that they all knew that using drug is dangerous and it could cause addiction, but none believed that it could happen to him/herself. The reality is that all of them, without exception, soon came to realize that physical dependence resulting from using drugs, just like Dawei's physical disability, was out of their own control. For his physical disability, Dawei found out that he had no way to control how he was perceived and treated by other people; for the physical dependence developed by using drugs, he and his addicted friends soon found out that they had lost control of their own bodies.

But drug addiction is more than physical dependence. It was in being with his friends, all losers in the social perception of society at large, that Dawei finally had someone that he could talk to, hang out with and have fun together. Dawei's parents both felt sorry for him after the accident caused his disability: they blamed it on their own fault of carelessness. "I could feel that they had been blaming themselves. They feel so sorry for me that they sometimes intentionally avoid me; they are afraid of talking to me. My relationship with my parents had been completely changed by the accident. We are no longer acting like son and parents, not in the traditional sense of Chinese culture. You know, even when I did something wrong, they did not dare to confront or criticize me. That is not usual, not what is supposed to happen between parents and children in Chinese families. Even when I decided to quit school, they did not say anything. I told them that I did not want to go to school any more, and then they agreed. Generally, there is no normal daily communication going on between my parents and me. I talk to my parents only when it is necessary; and they do the same to me." Dawei talked about his family relationship in a slow and mild manner. It was difficult for me to tell how he had been feeling about his parents over these years: hate, disappointment, or despair? But I could feel that something he did care about was missing in his family. He might have found what he wanted from his family among his relationship with "loser friends", other drug users; he finally had somewhere to go, someone to talk to, and some group he felt he belonged with and to.

I asked Dawei if he had ever hated the friend who brought drugs to him. He replied with a smile, "no, never. We are still friends. Nothing has really changed except that now we are patient friends," he burst into laughter. Many AIDS patients whom I met at the clinic knew each other for a long time. They had been friends even before they started using drugs together. They still kept each other as friends after they were diagnosed HIV positive, and they usually showed up together at the clinic for medication refills. I could tell that they were still friends. A nurse once made fun of them by saying, "you guys were duyou (drug friends) in the past and now you are bingyou (patient friends)." That is how Dawei learned the term "patient friends".

"We did it together. Nobody forced me to do it. There was none to blame." Dawei said, without even a little sense of regret. It was in being with his "loser friends", his drug friends that Dawei found the sense of belonging he needed and re-established his social networks, through which he was able to reconstruct and enjoy interpersonal relationships. It was the only way that Dawei and his friends could find to rebuild their own existential sense of living in the society.

In contrast to the popular belief, which has conceives of using drugs as absolutely self-destroying, Dawei and his friends were creating something that mattered much to themselves through using drugs together and sharing needles with each other.

I asked Dawei why he and his friends would share needles with each other. Dawei smiled, "it was not like what you think. We were sharing needles not because we could not afford extra needles or we were so eager to get the drug injection that we did not have time to get a new needle. It was not like that. We shared needles because we meant to do it. That was how we were supposed to do it. We were brothers. We used drugs together and shared needles with each other. It was nothing but brotherhood. That is what brothers should do." Here Dawei seems to allude to the ancient Chinese tradition of "blood brothers".

"Did you know that sharing needles could cause HIV infection?" I did not want to give up early on this issue.

"Yes, we knew that it could cause infection. But, at that time, we all thought that HIV/AIDS was still far away and there was no HIV/AIDS around among ourselves. So there was no need to worry about it."

"But it could also cause other infectious diseases, such as hepatitis. Weren't you afraid?"

"Yes. We knew that. But that's not the point. The point is that doing it together and sharing needles were exactly what we wanted. What matters most was not to get the drug, but to use it together and share with each other. That is the point." Dawei looked at me for seconds, and then with a smile coming to his face, he turned away to look out the window. "You won't understand it," he added.

Dawei's expression reminded me of the way Jun said "you people". I believed that Dawei and Jun both had the same feeling at the similar moment: how could you people understand us?

I found myself not completely convinced by Dawei's excessively romantic way of reframing his experience of using drugs; but I could not deny that using drugs and sharing needles with drug friends did provide him what he was looking for but had never found elsewhere: The sense of belonging, the sense of living with social networks and interpersonal relationships, the sense of being a normal person rather than being categorized as a cripple or loser, and the sense of not being stigmatized.

Contrary to Dawei's romantic narrative, his mother presented me with another image meant to express the suffering, stress and stigma that Dawei, as both a drug user and an AIDS patient, had brought to his family. I met Dawei's mother several times at the clinic when she accompanied him to the clinic for medication refills. She was around 50 but looked much older. From her grey hair, weary look and the outdated dress style, I could tell at my first sight of her that she had been through a lot.

While Dawei was receiving a regular medical test, I had a short talk with his mother. Our conversation inevitably started with Dawei's disability. The mother repeated the story of the accident. In the end, she sighed, "My husband and I just felt that we owe him a lot. There was nothing we could do to take back what we did to him. You know what it means to people who have disabilities. They are waste people in other's eyes.

But you could do nothing about it. You have to deal with it alone; as his parents, we have to deal with it by ourselves." The mother stopped to wipe tears away.

"Because of the accident, we both felt that we owe him. So we basically let him do whatever he wants to do. We just don't want to make him upset. We know that he has been living under great pressure. He has never had many friends, never had a girlfriend. As his parents, we have the obligation to take care of him; given his disability, we have every reason to do that, even take care of him for the rest of his life, if we can live that long."

"How did your son quit school?" I asked.

"He told us that he didn't want to go to school any more. My husband and I both felt that it might not be a correct decision. But what could we do? Even if he could have finished high school, or even go to college, what would he get? Who will give a job to a disabled person like him? Even a lot of healthy people cannot find a job today; we have no reason to believe that he can do better. So we just agreed to his request of quitting school. After that, we tried to find him something to do. But it was not easy."

"So he has never worked?"

"No. He just stayed at home. You know, at the time, my husband and I had to work. We had no idea what he had been doing for those days when we were not home. He often locked himself in his room even when we were home. Sometimes he prepared food if he wanted. He had a few friends, sometimes he went out with them. We didn't ask whom he was with and what they were doing together; he didn't tell us either. It was in those days that he learned using drug from those friends. It is my guess afterwards. We had no idea about it until he was caught using drugs by the police."

The mother believed that Dawei learned using drugs from bad friends. The bad thing has to be learned from bad friends. Generally, many parents believe in their children's innocence and attribute children's misbehavior and wrongdoing to the bad friends they made, though the children might not have the same view.

"It was his friends who did this to him. Later I found out that most of his friends are losers who quit school, have no jobs, wander in the streets all the time and have nothing to do. They are basically idlers. You can tell what he could learn from those people. Nothing good but bad! They are just the dregs of society."

The mother felt angry with her son's bad friends, but she had never blamed her own son. "He is still my son, no matter what he had done. It was his friends who should be blamed for this. They should go to jail. Look at what they have done to my son." The mother will never blame her son, but her work unit didn't let this go so easily.

After Dawei was caught using drugs, the police sent him to a local detox center under the required detoxification policy, which was launched in China in the 1980s. According to this policy, addicts who are caught using drugs are compelled to enter detox centers to receive involuntary detoxification. The detox centers are controlled and managed by public security bureaus. During their stay at the centers, addicts are forced to receive medication and psychiatric treatment. In addition, they are compelled to do physical labor and participate in law and moral education classes in order to remove their physical and psychological dependence on drugs. Later during my field work in Dexin, I had a chance to visit the local detox center located in a mountain far away from the city. The center was managed as a quasi-prison. It was divided into two sections: the mandatory camp and the volunteer camp. The former is for the addicts who are caught by the police; the volunteer camp is for the addicts who are brought in by their families.

The message that Dawei was caught using drugs and sent to the detox center was officially delivered to his family and also his parents' work units. His father and mother were both criticized in public at their respective work units. What does the parents' work unit have to do with their son's drug problem? It has to be understood in the context of the Chinese danwei (work unit) system. In China, a work unit is the name given to a state-owned enterprise. During the planned economy period prior to market economic reforms a work unit acted as a communist party controlled hierarchical system that monitored every aspect of all members' lives. Workers were bound to their work units for their whole lives. Each danwei provided housing, food, even child care, schooling, and hospitalization for its own members. A work unit had a substantial and profound influence on the lives of its members, who had to obtain permission from the work unit for marriage and having children, sometimes even for buying a bicycle. A work unit was managed not only as a place of employment, but also as the principal site where Party policies and moral education are implemented. Members who did not comply with Party policies could be punished by their work units: the leaders of a danwei might teach them a lesson via private talk, or criticize them in public in open meeting, decrease their salary, withhold the incentives they were promised, even remove their positions.

When the market economic reforms were launched in the late 1980s, many social services provided within danwei, such as child care, schools, and clinics, were removed in the face of increasing competition from private enterprises and foreign companies. The control of work units over their members was greatly weakened. However, the work unit still can exert power in today's China. The effort that the government has made to maintain its control of individuals through danwei has been weakened but really never ended. That is why Dawei's parents were criticized by their work units for their son's drug abuse.

"It was so embarrassing." Dawei's mother said when she recalled the meeting. The leader, party secretary, of her work unit mentioned her name in front of all of her workmates and blamed her for carelessness in teaching her son. "He said that it was my husband and I that should be blamed for the fact that my son became an addict and my family must take all the responsibilities. He questioned me in front of all the people in the meeting. He asked me how I could let it happen. I didn't know what to say. It was so embarrassing. And then he went on to say that my family brought shame to this work unit and damaged the work unit's good image and reputation, and it was all because of my son. I felt so ashamed at the moment; I really hoped that there was a hole in the ground so I could hide myself inside or escape from there. It was diu si ren le (literally losing face to death)." The mother started shaking her head while she went on, "I just felt that I don't have the face (lian) to face anyone."

"Then what about your husband?"

"The same. He was criticized too in a meeting in his work unit. In addition, the leaders demanded that he write a jiantao (a self-criticism report) and then submit it to the Party secretary. After that, we felt so ashamed that we didn't even have the courage to raise our heads in front of our workmates."

Criticism in a public meeting, I believe, is part of the historical remains of struggle sessions. Struggle sessions, well known as one of the methods applied to foster class struggle during the Chinese Cultural Revolution (1966–1976), were originally applied in rural Chinese areas by the Communist Party from the late 1930s to the 1940s in order to launch rural revolution: turning poor peasants against landlords and other people who were not on the side of the Communist Party. Struggle sessions were so organized that they narrated the suffering caused by the exploiting class, morally categorized members of that class as belonging to bad elements, attacked these class enemies, confiscated their properties, and mobilized peasants' support for revolution. During the Chinese Cultural Revolution, in the name of class struggle, struggle sessions were used to achieve personal ends: seeking political power, eliminating personal enemies, or simply protecting oneself from becoming the object of struggle by turning the spotlight on others.

Humiliating, accusing, and attacking are the major techniques applied in struggle sessions. In today's China, the extremely radical and violent form of struggle sessions is gone, but the idea behind this political technique and certain milder methods, such as humiliation and criticism, remain for implementing social control. That is what happened to Dawei's parents. The detox center informed the family and their work units about Dawei's drug problem, and then the parents were both criticized at the work unit's meeting. Informing the family and the work unit results from the absence of the idea of personal privacy in China; but the key to understand this official procedure lies in recognizing it is meant to have one's misconduct known by others, to humiliate and stigmatize the offender and his family, to damage their moral status, to punish them socially, and also to warn others.

The concepts of human rights and personal privacy in the western perspective might not be robust in China; but that does not mean these concepts are completely absent in China. In fact, the fact that the idea of face has played a significant role throughout Chinese culture proves that Chinese people have their own indigenous views of human rights and personal privacy. The condition can be put this way: one has to be a person rather than a non-person in order to have the right to ask for one's human rights and personal privacy. For the disabled, gay men, drug users, or HIV/AIDS patients, who are not considered to be normal persons, they are believed not to be qualified for human rights and personal privacy. In other words, human rights and personal privacy in Chinese culture are a particularistic rather than universalistic idea. Or we can say, in the Chinese context, human rights or personal privacy are not the perspective or discourse to be applied when it comes to non-persons.

As a matter of fact, humiliation and stigmatization have been used as major methods in fighting the drug problem and HIV/AIDS epidemic. Stigmatization has been widely applied in many areas for social control and it has been widely believed to be an effective prevention measure. That is to say, using humiliation and stigmatization as social punishment to frighten people away from socially defined misconduct, such as sexual deviance and illicit drug use; while informing the family and work unit is the usual way to proceed. In March 2006, the Law on Public Security Administration Punishments issued by the Ministry of Public Security states that people who are caught visiting prostitutes shall be held in detention for 10–15 days with a fine up to 5,000 yuan; if the circumstances are minor, the offenders shall be detained up to five days with a fine up to 500 yuan (Article 66); if the offenders are held in detention, their families shall be informed (Article 97). A big debate occurred over the issue of "informing family" after the law was published. People who questioned it argued that informing family breaks the offender's human right and personal privacy; they were afraid that informing the family might directly cause family conflict and result in divorce; they also suspected that the public security system is trying to aggravate punishment by informing the offender's family; while the public security spokesman clarified that families have the right to know why the offenders are held in detention and informing the family is a law procedure rather than a punishment. The spokesman also insisted that informing the family is an obligatory legal procedure and that the work unit should be informed when the family is not available. Many people agreed that informing the family is a much better way than detention or fine to scare potential offenders away from visiting prostitutes; they also believe that it is a far more effective punishment than detention or fine to prevent offenders from repeating it again. Some people took this procedure seriously as a method of preventing sexual deviance and considered it helpful in stopping the spread of the HIV/AIDS epidemic. The debate over the law revealed what informing family means in Chinese daily life; moreover, the debate was not mainly focused on the offender's human rights or personal privacy, although this issue has been voiced; instead, it was all about what telling the family could do to the offenders, the potential damage that it could cause to family and marriage, and also whether it could be misused by police as an aggravated punishment. This example shows how humiliation and stigmatization have been perceived in daily life and how they can be, or have been applied in legal practice of China.

In Dawei's case, we can observe how humiliation was used to stigmatize drug users and their families in order to mobilize and promote the social anti-drug campaign, which was called the People's Anti-drug War. In the case of HIV/AIDS, many Chinese health professionals agreed that humiliation and stigmatization are helpful in dealing with HIV/AIDS epidemic. According to Dr. Meng in Beijing, a health expert from Thailand once mentioned to him that the future of China in fighting HIV/AIDS is much more promising than the situation faced by Thailand because of the great shame associated with sexual deviance in Chinese culture, which is absent in Thailand. It can help prevent the HIV/AIDS epidemic. Although Dr. Meng had to admit that in today's China the shame connected to sexual deviance might not be as strong as it was in the past, he did believe that shame is still an important factor that the country can count on in preventing the HIV/AIDS epidemic from escalating.

The stigma associated with using drugs took up a large part of my conversation with Dawei's mother. In contrast to Dawei's romantic narrative of his experience of using drugs and sharing needles, his drug problem was socially categorized and defined as personal moral deviance, a danger to the society, and shame for his family and their networks. Since my research was supposed to focus on the stigma associated with HIV/AIDS, I went on to ask Dawei's mother about her family's experience after Dawei tested HIV positive.

"Look at what we had been through. Do you think that we still have anything left to lose? No, we already lost everything and we had nothing to lose. We had nothing to lose at all. Compared to Dawei's disability and drug problem, HIV/AIDS was indeed bad news to our family. But it could not make things even worse because we were already in the worst situation before that day," his mother said with a bitter smile on her face.

"We already lost all of our face because of my son's drug problem; we could not lose any more because there was nothing left. So there was no need to worry about it."

"Does your work unit know about your son's HIV/AIDS status?"

"I don't really know that. Indeed I don't care anymore. My husband and I are already retired. We don't have to go to work units to look at other people's faces. Once you lost everything; you simply don't care much how you look in other people's eyes."

"Then what about your family's relatives?"

"We haven't contacted each other for a long time. Since Dawei was found using drugs, we stopped visiting each other as we did before except for big festivals. We are afraid of seeing them; they are also afraid of contacting us. We both try to avoid each other. That is it."

Dawei's mother seemed to have run out of energy and didn't have much to say about what happened after Dawei contracted AIDS; she was exhausted by narrating the family story which had already exhausted her real life by what had already happened to her family before she learned of Dawei's HIV/AIDS. For her, Dawei's HIV/AIDS is not a new problem to her family but part of never-ending disasters that are a continuum of the same family tragedy. For the family, the stigma associated with HIV/AIDS is not perceived as a new and separate issue; instead, it is considered in the entirety of the painful life experience to which the stigma associated with disability, drug problem and HIV/AIDS have contributed. Stigma constitutes a total family experience of being isolated and discriminated, but as this indicates the sources of stigma are many, not just HIV/AIDS.

Shuanglong — He Is Not My Son Anymore

In contrast to Dawei's humility, Shuanglong seemed more talkative and always showed cynicism toward almost everything. He was in his late 20s, short and swarthy. Shuanglong admitted that he started using drugs after he quit high school when he was around 15.

"I was not the kind of student who fit in at school. And I believe that school is not the only way that you can make a life. So I just quit." Shuanglong said with a smile of never-minding anything. I asked him how he started using drugs. With the same smile on his face, he said, "Nothing special. I had several friends, and we always kept each other company after quitting school. And we tried this stuff together for fun. And it was fun." It seemed that my question brought Shuanglong back to his happy old days. He looked up at the ceiling, with the permanent smile on his face.

"What exactly did you feel when you were using drugs?"

"You just feel nothing but good things. You will see anything you want appearing right in front of you. I mean anything you can imagine. When you get high, you can feel it and it is so real for you. You can even touch it. There will be no trouble, nothing that you have to worry about every day. Anything you can imagine will come true."

"Then what about after that?"

"Hah, everything is still the same as it was. It is like waking up from a beautiful dream. But, at least, you had one moment that you could get away from those troubling things."

"Then what had been troubling you?"

Shuanglong sighed, looking down at the floor, "A lot of things."

"Tell me about it. You don't seem to be the kind of person who worries much. That was the impression you gave me."

Shuanglong looked around with an awkward smile this time, trying to find something to look at. "A lot of things. It is hard to tell," Shuanglong would not go deep into this issue. I decided to change the topic and turned to ask him how he and his friends used to find drugs. "They could be found everywhere if you had connections. And it was really cheap. You could buy a gram of heroin for 30–50 yuan in the 1990s."

I recalled that when I was wandering on Foreigners Street in the old town of Dexin, I often ran into several old ladies who were trying to sell me something. But they spoke the local Bai language, of which I could not understand a single word at the time. Later I was told by my local friends that they were selling drugs, often to foreign tourists. I mentioned this to Shuanglong; he smiled, saying, "That is not heroin, just marijuana or opium made in nearby mountain areas."

"Are you still using drugs?"

Shuanglong shook his head and replied, "No, no, I have not used drugs for a long time." He looked at me and smiled.

In following interviews, I was able to continue my conversation with Shuanglong. I asked Shuanglong if he knew sharing needles with other drug users could cause HIV infection. He said that he had no idea about it; and then went on to complain about the government's not telling people about this danger.

"We didn't know anything about HIV/AIDS. We thought that it only existed in foreign countries and there was no HIV/AIDS in China. If I had known it, I would not have been infected. So it was the government's fault that caused my disease. They didn't tell us. The government is the one to blame."

"When did you find out that you were infected?"

"Actually, I was caught using drugs in 2000 and sent to the local detox center where they gave me the HIV/AIDS test. But they did not tell me about this test; they didn't tell me the test results either. Later when I got out of the center and became very sick in 2002, I was hospitalized, and then I tested HIV positive. That was the first time I was informed that I had AIDS. But I was told that I was found HIV positive 2 years before when I was held at the detox center. Those people working at the detox center already knew it 2 years before, and they kept my test records, but they never told me about it."

It was the first time I heard that the detox center hid the HIV/AIDS status from the drug users under their control. Later I asked several other patients about this issue and found out that it was true. I assumed that it was another case of information control techniques for which the Chinese government has been criticized: it often responds this way to danger and threat: hiding the truth from the general population in order not to turn the danger and threat against its own authority. But this is a different case. It is not hiding the truth from the general population but hiding the disease from the patients themselves. Later I talked to Dr. Wang about the detox center's concealing the HIV/AIDS test results from patients. He gave me another explanation from a more practical perspective. "The detox center chose not to tell patients because they were afraid that once those drug users knew their HIV/AIDS status for the first time, they might become very upset and could intentionally have other inmates infected. It was not only a danger to the other inmates held at the center but also a threat to the management of the center. It could cause the spread of HIV/AIDS epidemic within the center. So the center chose not to tell them in order to protect other inmates and maintain the normal management of the center." I argued that the patients had the right to know about their condition; in addition they could have started seeking treatment in time if they had known their situation earlier. Dr. Wang replied, "That could be right. But the reality is much more complicated. In that context, it is no longer an individual thing; instead it becomes an issue related to the broader community and even society. You have to consider the whole situation in the perspective of the society rather than deal with it as an individual problem."

I suggested that the detox center could have released the HIV infected drug users and put them under the care of hospitals if they were afraid that these patients might endanger the other inmates. Dr. Wang said, "At that time we didn't have enough resources to deal with the HIV/AIDS epidemic if the detox center sent everyone they found infected to us. Even today we are still short of all kinds of resources, including manpower, equipment and funding. More important is the policy issue. We are working under the rules made in terms of the government's policies. We, including my clinic and the detox center, do what we are told to do. We don't create policies ourselves. If there are no policies, no rules, we can do nothing about it. The HIV/AIDS epidemic is still new to the whole country, even today we are still learning how to deal with it."

The concern of social security, the absence of necessary resources, the government's lack of experience, institutions, and policies in the face of the HIV/AIDS epidemic all have contributed to compromise the human rights of HIV/AIDS patients like Shuanglong. Violating human rights and the practice of sacrificing some people in order to save the rest and maintain general social order are not rare cases at all in China's battle with the HIV/AIDS epidemic. It is easy for anyone to criticize all this misconduct from the perspective of human rights; however, for Dr. Wang who is working on the front lines fighting the HIV/AIDS epidemic, the misconduct approved by the government and practiced by various institutions seemed to be appropriate and necessary. But it did reveal the dilemma and urgency faced by the whole country in dealing with a new epidemic. In the face of this dilemma, what matters most might not be what should be done but what could be done with the existing resources and the sense of what really mattered more.

However, the dilemma constituted in the local context cannot be used as an excuse to justify misconduct. The suffering caused by this damaging approach to people like Shuanglong and their families cannot be denied. Nor can it be simply waved away as the fault of society or the government, albeit they matter. Blame needs to be shared with particular programs, people, and policy implementation.

During my later conversation with Shuanglong, he told me that his father's death is related to his using drugs. When Shuanglong was caught using drugs, his parents, just like Dawei's parents, were also criticized in a public meeting at their work units. His father was a low-level cadre at his work unit and used to have a good reputation among his workmates. Shortly after being criticized in the meeting, the father died of a heart attack. Being a cadre of the work unit, who was expected to be a moral example, he simply could not stand being humiliated and died of anger and shame. Although he used to suffer his heart disease and high blood pressure, according to Shuanglong, his sudden death was definitely associated with the criticism session held at his work unit.

During the Cultural Revolution, more than 7 million people were estimated to have been killed or committed suicide because of the unbearable attacks and humiliation caused by struggle sessions (Rummel 1991). The number of suicide was believed up to 200,000. Although the exact number of deaths has never been released by the Chinese government, some numbers can be found in local documents. In 1968, in Changchun, a city in northeast China, among 1,929 people who died in struggle sessions from May to December, 184 were killed and 1,745 committed suicide (*Changchun gonganzhi*, p. 267); in Hunan Province, 326 people committed suicide in Nandao county from August to October, 1967; in Lingling district, 1,397 people committed suicide because of struggle session (*Dashidai wenzhai*, July 1997). These numbers show how serious stress and suffering could be caused by accusing, attacking and humiliating a person during struggle sessions. Although the scale and degree of the criticism session that Shuanglong's father participated in could not even come close to the experience during the Cultural Revolution, it approved to result in his sudden death from a heart attack. However, in the public narrative, it was Shuanglong rather than the work unit or the criticism session that was revealed as the cause of his father's death. Even Shuanglong himself believed that he made his father angry to death. From that time, Shuanglong became not only a loser who quit school and had no job and a drug user who was killing himself, but also a son who had killed his father. A heavy burden indeed!

After Shuanglong's family was informed that he was caught using drugs, his parents got very angry with him; they blamed him for having done nothing but harm to the family. They attributed Shuanglong's quitting school and unemployment to his irresponsibility and failure to uphold his family. They blamed him for not studying hard enough at school; they blamed him for not trying hard enough to find a job; they blamed him for lacking a sense of family; they blamed him for being so selfish that he had never considered how to support the family but always taken what he wanted from the family; they blamed him for having never considered how to repay his parents for taking care of him but only bringing more and more troubles to them. In his parents' eyes, Shuanglong, as a drug user, became a waste person or even a parasite to his family. When his father died shortly after the criticism session held at his work unit, Shuanglong became an enemy to his family.

Shuanglong recalled those days, saying, "My mother shouted at me, 'why don't you just leave! How could you still have the face to come back to this family? What kind of son are you? You even had your father killed. Get out of my house!' I also felt guilty and didn't have the courage to stay at home. So I had to leave and stay at one of my friend's places for a while. Later when I went back home, my mother would not stop blaming me or shouting at me. When she really stopped, she started crying and complaining, 'what have we done to make you do this to us? Do we owe you anything?' There was nothing I could say. I just had to endure it."

Given the fact that using drugs has been considered a crime one commits to his/her own family, drug users are often criticized as non-persons who have no sense of family, do not care for anyone but themselves, always tell lies and cheat on family members for money to buy drugs, and even steal from their own families. Before I left Beijing for Dexin, Zhanshan at the AIDS Care Center once warned me to be careful about working with drug users. He said, "Those drug users are not like us. They never tell truth and always lie. You won't hear anything trustworthy from them. They are all liars and cheaters. Don't trust them. They can do anything to their own families in order to get drugs. Can you imagine that? How could a person wave a knife to their parents and threaten them for money to spend on drugs?" Based on his own experience, Zhanshan gave me his views of drug users. He described drug users as the worst type of persons, which conforms to the image of drug users presented in public media: the most despised persons who don't care for their own families and even do harm to their own family members. Such persons are considered non-persons, even worse than beasts (qinshou buru) because they have no sense of renqing (moral relationships) at all (butong renqing). In Chinese culture, renqing is the basic and most important idea of being a person. It means that a person should recognize and care for various interpersonal relationships, locate his/her own position in the local social networks, know how to act in different relationships, have a sense of returning a favor in an appropriate way. Among various interpersonal relationships, family relations are the most important and valued; family relationships and family members are the last ones that a person has to care about even if he/she has to ignore other relationships or relatives under certain circumstances. Therefore, a person who has no sense of family and does not care about family will be despised as a non-person who does not deserve any sympathy no matter what happen to him/her. In that case, if families decide to abandon the non-persons or do anything to punish them, they will not be criticized because non-persons are considered to deserve nothing better.

Two cases of law case will be quoted in order to reveal what the idea of renqing really means in the Chinese culture and how it is perceived and applied even when this core moral reality conflicts with the practice of law in the local world.

In 2005, a father killed his 36-year-old son in Sichuan Province (*Huaxi dushibao*, September 21, 2005). His son was a village scourge. Every time when he got drunk, he would beat anyone he ran into in the village. Late one night, the son was drunk again. When he arrived home, he started beating his younger brother without any reason. The father came out of his room to stop him, but the son turned to beat his father. Out of the anger accumulated over years, the father ran into the kitchen, grabbed a knife, and then killed his son. Having witnessed his father's murder, the younger son was shocked. But the 73-year-old father said in a calm manner, "Today I got rid of this scourge. We don't have to endure this anymore. It is over." When police arrived at the crime scene, many villagers expressed their sympathy with the father and spoke in defense of him. They told police that the victim was such an evil man that he did not deserve any sympathy. "Nobody would care if he was killed. I have never seen a husband like him beating his wife so badly. He even beat his father. Is he still a human? He was really worse than beasts." Having received the shocking news, the victim's wife came back home from another city where she was working. The wife cried for the family tragedy rather than her husband's death. She said, "I don't feel sad for him at all. He used to beat me up almost every day. He also beat his own parents. He deserves it." After the old man was arrested, the villagers sent a jointly signed letter to the local justice department, expressing their support and asking for a less severe punishment.

In 2007, a mother poisoned her son to death in a village of Chongqing (Chongqing chenbao, July 10, 2007). The son was well known as a ruffian in the village. He not only beat other villagers anytime he wanted but also often beat his father and caused his father's blindness. Finally, the mother could not live with her son's evil conduct anymore; she put poison in his food and killed him. The family tragedy resulted in a murder case: a mother killed her evil son. After the mother was arrested, more than 160 villagers jointly signed a letter and sent it to the local judge who was on the case. In the letter, the villagers defended the mother and asked for her release. They spoke of the mother's murder of her own son as a brave and unselfish action of weiminchuhai (ridding the people of a scourge). Although the judge insisted that there was no doubt it was a murder case, he could not ignore the great social pressure and had to consider the villagers' appeal. In the end, the judge waived the death sentence and sentenced the mother to prison for five years.

The two cases reveal how people perceive the evil sons who had no sense of renqing and how they feel about the facts that two non-persons were punished and even killed by their own families. People expressed their sympathy to the killers rather than the victims; they attributed the sense of renqing to the parents who killed their own evil sons.

Renqing, as one of the basic ideas constituting the local moral sense in the Chinese daily life, is the key to understand what really matters, what is perceived as right or wrong and also how a person is evaluated and judged in the Chinese local world. Having or not having the sense of renqing determines whether or not a person should be considered and treated as a real person or a non-person; for people who already lost the sense of renqing, it is believed morally right to treat them as non-persons: despising, discriminating, stigmatizing, punishing, even killing them without any mercy or sympathy. In this sense, stigmatization is the embodiment and application of the local moral sense.

For Shuanglong, in the local moral sense, he betrayed and abandoned his family by using drugs and causing his father's death; his misconduct showed that he had no sense of renqing, which was why he became a non-person in the local view. Since he became a non-person, the detox center believed that they had the right to ignore his basic human rights and violate his privacy at ease. Moreover, it was because of his identity as a non-person that the detox center felt it right to inform his parents' work units about his drug problem; that the work units thought they had the right to hold a criticism session and criticize his parents in public without caring about their face. Shuanglong's identity as a non-person had been transferred to his family and thus his family's moral face was damaged too. Hence, the work units and other people felt it right not to care about their moral status anymore; there would be no risk to humiliate and stigmatize the whole family. Stigmatization is believed the morally right thing to do to non-persons.

When I asked Shuanglong about the situation after he was found out to be HIV positive, he got lost and confused, "Look at what I had been through and had gone through so far, do you still think it will make any difference?" Shuanglong seemed to have difficulty in marking a clear dividing line in his life experience between before and after he had contracted AIDS. For him, such a time point might not even have existed. His experience after he contracted AIDS might not have appeared so different for him from what he had experienced before that; instead, it was the same. He had always been despised, discriminated and stigmatized. For Shuanglong, his experience of suffering has never changed from one phase to another; it just kept growing and accumulating. As Dawei said, HIV/AIDS neither added anything new to his life nor made it even worse because things were already in the worst situation, and his life had always been in the worst situation. For Dawei and Shuanglong, the suffering resulting from being stigmatized did not start from the day they contracted AIDS; instead, it began much earlier than that day: It started since Dawei became disabled, since they quit school and could not find jobs, since they wandered around with "bad" friends, since they began using drugs. Stigma has never stopped hunting them; they have always been living with stigma. That is why they did not feel much difference about the stigma associated with HIV/AIDS and why they usually felt lost when it came to focusing especially on the stigma associated with just HIV/AIDS.

Dawei and Shuanglong are not the only exceptions. Among the patients who contracted AIDS through sharing needles, I found it very common that they often appeared to have relatively clear memories about what happened to them after they were found using drugs; contrarily, most of them spoke little about what happened after they were found to be HIV positive. Given the fact that these patients who all had long-term life experiences of being stigmatized for various reasons, the stigma associated with HIV/AIDS means nothing new to them and might not constitute a strong stimulus for them to remember or discuss. However, there is a second possible explanation: they did remember, but they did not want to talk about it. The question is why these patients would rather talk about being stigmatized because of using drugs than talk about being stigmatized because of HIV/AIDS. My hypothesis is that HIV/AIDS, compared to using drugs, is more deeply involved in being stigmatized within the family. In China, owing to the feeling of shame, people generally are reluctant to disclose how they are mistreated within families, especially not to someone outside the family, though they are more willing to speak about how they are treated unjustly by institutions or people outside their families. According to Dawei and Shuanglong's narratives, drug users are already strongly stigmatized within families: they are blamed, criticized, and discriminated against as non-persons by their own families. Could the stigma associated with HIV/AIDS make the situation even worse?

My answer is yes, but for these patients and their families the difference is one of degree, not of nature.

Deng *et al.* (2007) conducted a research onut stigma related to drug abuse and HIV/AIDS in a Dai ethnic group in Yunnan Province. They described in detail how the drug users are stigmatized in the local context. They pointed out that stigmatization and discrimination were "manifested in all contexts and all aspects of the drug abusers' life" (2007: 1566). The following is quoted from their research article:

"Within the family, the use of separate tableware and dining was a common practice. Although parents did not reject their drug-taking children, they treated them differently because of distrust and dislike" (2007: 1566).

"The common jobs they (drug abusers) could get were inferior ones, with low pay and discriminatory treatment, such as casual farmhands or restaurant helpers and janitors. Separate tableware and dining were common practices in the workplace as well. The tableware used by drug abusers had to be sterilized or discarded after use" (2007: 1567).

"In the community context, drug abusers were excluded from weddings, festivals, funerals, and religious activities. Although there were no written rules against drug abusers' participation in such activities, they rarely attended them because they were looked down upon by others and no one would share a table with heroin abusers" (2007: 1567).

When drug abusers died, "they (their families) still held or attended traditional funeral ceremonies for heroin abusers. However, no one, not even family members, was willing to touch the corpse or carry the coffin. According to the ritual, the corpse must be washed and wrapped in calico before being put in the coffin. The death of a heroin abuser was considered ill-omened, not only because most drug abusers were aged under 60 years, but also because they had died from deviant behavior. People were fearful of getting bad luck from heroin abusers" (2007: 1567). The family had to hire other drug abusers to do it. "Moreover, the drug abuser's body could not be buried in the ancestral grave yard. Instead, a separate but an inferior place was designated for them in case their evil spirits would influence ancestors and offspring" (2007: 1567).

"Death was perceived as the only relief for drug abusers and family members. Neither parents nor spouses felt sad about the death of a heroin abuser. On the contrary, most respondents used the words 'free', 'easy', 'happy' and 'unattached' to describe their feelings about the death of a drug abuser. Although it is customary for the Dai people to throw away the belongings of the dead, under normal circumstances family members still kept some valuable mementos as keepsakes. However, many family members reported that they discarded everything that had been used or touched by a heroin abuser in order to 'throw away all the bad luck'. The room where the drug abusers lived had then to be emptied and locked up" (2007: 1567).

"Drug abusers were also stigmatized in the institutional contexts … Drug abuse was a new phenomenon in the community, and it was condemned by the religion because of its associated deviant behaviors, such as stealing, cheating, and drug trafficking. Drug abuse was viewed as an individual choice but not a fate, and hence the drug abusers were considered to deserve the consequences of their actions" (2007: 1567–1568).

"To the Dai people, the community is one big family that should be respected, maintained and protected by all community members. However, heroin abusers became destructive to the community because the addiction drove them into immoral practices, such as stealing, cheating, and drug trafficking. Such immoral behaviors disrupted the 'family' system. Hence, drug abusers were not only punished with written and unwritten social regulations but also isolated from the big 'family'. Additionally, in combination with the local beliefs surrounding illness and death, the association between drug abuse and HIV/AIDS was another source of stigmatization" (2007: 1568).

"While illness was considered as part of normal life, those who could not recover from prolonged sickness and who suffered acute diseases were thought to be bewitched, and their death was a portentous one. Drug abusers with HIV/AIDS fit well into this category. The existing social stratification by age and gender in the community was also reflected in individuals' and community's responses to drug abusers and PLHA (people living with HIV/AIDS). While all drug abusers were 'condemned', older persons were more likely to be forgiven. Female drug abusers would be even more stigmatized than male abusers, but women infected by their drug abusing husbands received great sympathy" (2007: 1568).

"Discrimination was also legitimated in the form of policies and community strategies for controlling heroin abuse. For example, drug abusers were imprisoned in DATCs (detox centers) for detoxification and rehabilitation for 3 or 6 months. However, if they could not quit drugs or refuse to return to the DATC, they would be jailed for three or eight years. Anyone who became a drug abuser would have their private fields confiscated for the public treasury; be deprived of their civil rights; be dismissed from youth groups; and be fined 200 RMB (Renminbi or Yuan) if they stole in the community. Villagers were not allowed to buy anything from heroin abusers and would be fined 200–300 RMB if they received or accommodated any foreign drug dealers and abusers" (2007: 1568).

Similar to the general belief that the HIV/AIDS patient is sentenced to the penalty of social death, a common fact that drug users seldom quit using drugs makes people believe that they are also morally dead. Especially when families have to witness, endure and suffer the never-ending episodes of detoxification and relapse, they often end up running out of family finance for detoxification and treatment, losing hope for a complete recovery, and feeling exhausted from shame and humiliation. Drug users become a common object of family hatred and isolation. They are not considered family members anymore; instead, their families simply wish that they had never come to be part of the family. In this sense, both HIV/AIDS and drug abuse relapse mean the same thing to families: there is no cure for the disease or for the person. The HIV/AIDS patients and drug users become a family burden that their families wish they could get rid of rather than family members who deserve concern and sympathy.

Ware *et al.* (2005) point out that stereotyping, as a medium for stigmatization, might have contributed to unequal treatment for drug users and other populations living with HIV. Although their research results "revealed stability and control as well as chaos in the lives of study participants; frequency of drug use varied considerably; using did interfere with adherence, but not in every circumstance or all cases" (2005: 565). However, medical professionals generally assume that "drug users are less capable than others of adhering to complicated medication regimens" (2005: 565). They believe "(1) drug users lead chaotic lives; (2) active drug users are always using drugs; (3) being under the influence of drugs precludes taking medications as prescribed; and (4) drug users are intrinsically different from non-users in the lives they lead and the problems they face" (2005: 565). As I have observed in my field work, the Chinese medical professionals also perceive the drug users the same way: they are not trustworthy.

Drug abuse relapse seemed very common among the patients whom I met in Dexin. Many patients, even when they were on anti-viral treatment for AIDS, had never stopped using drugs, though they often admitted it. A few of them admitted it when nurses and I tried to talk with them on this issue in private. Later, with the helpful hints from nurses I could even tell whether or not a patient just used drugs before he or she came to the clinic. Sometimes when they came in with a listless face, they kept silent and acted slowly; but there were several times when they showed up happy with red cheeks, they became so talkative and excited that they could hardly sit down. The explanation had to be that they just used drugs and they were feeling a high. Sometimes when I handed patients the money for their participation in the research, I asked myself what if they were going to buy drugs right after they left the clinic. I was not sure if the money was helping or hurting them.

One day, I went to the clinic and found a middle-aged woman talking aloud. Dr. Wang introduced the woman, Shuanglong's mother, to me and then told me that Shuanglong was caught using drugs again. Shuanglong was caught by the police and sent to the local detox center. Since Shuanglong was going to be held in the center for several months and we were unable to have his electronic medication bottle scanned during that period, he had to be removed from the research program. At the beginning, I thought Shuanglong's mother was asking Dr. Wang for a favor to help Shuanglong since Dr. Wang's clinic had a close working relationship with the detox center. But I soon found out that she was not. She kept blaming Shuanglong for unfilialness and complaining how much she had suffered from that unfilialness.

Dr. Wang appeared angry with this situation. He blamed Shuanglong's mother, "how could you let this happen? How have you been taking care of your son? He was using drugs while receiving treatment for AIDS. The anti-viral medication is provided by the government for free. Do you have any idea about that? Do you have any idea how much those medications cost the government? You guys just do not care, do you? It is such a waste."

She said she was sorry to Dr. Wang at first, and then stated that that was not what she meant. "I have not minded his (Shuanglong) business since a long time ago. He is no longer my son. I don't recognize this son. How could I still consider him my son? Look at what he has done to my family? He is so unfilial. He even got his father killed. As a mother I think I have done what I should have done. I gave him food, clothes, money, and a place to sleep. I have been taking care of him for so many years; I think I have done enough. As a mother, I have done enough. I don't have any regret. I have always observed my obligation to him as a mother to her son, but what about him? What did he do to me, to the family? Has he ever thought about this family? Has he ever thought about how to repay his parents? I already gave up on him. I have done enough; no matter what is going to happen to him, it is not my business anymore. I don't care. I won't care anymore. He has nothing to do with me."

The mother was so very upset. She was standing at the doorway of a clinic room. While she was talking, she kept crossing the door line to walk in or out. When she talked to Dr. Wang, she walked in a little, facing toward Dr. Wang; while talking about her son, she would retreat, stand right outside the door, and then face the door or the outside. It was as if she was talking to nobody. She did not have the courage to face anyone when she was speaking of her son. "I felt so shamed. We were running out of our money because of him. But that was not the end yet. He lost face for the whole family, made me and his father humiliated. We just feel that we are losing face to death. We have no face anymore at all. It is such a shame."

In the end, the mother turned to ask Dr. Wang not to bother to mind Shuanglong's business anymore. She expressed her regret about the troubles that Shuanglong had made for Dr. Wang and also her appreciation for Dr. Wang's help in the past. She said, "I already gave up on him; you, Dr. Wang, don't have to care him anymore either. I believe that you also have done what you could have done to help him. He will not quit using drugs until death. If he does not want to live anymore, so be it."

The mother continued to criticize her son for unfilialness. She marked a dividing line between herself and her son. Her narratives showed how a family feels about the drug users and HIV/AIDS patient within. Her statement that her son had nothing to do with her indicated that these patients are categorized as non-persons who have no sense of family connection and filiality. They are not identified by their own families as members anymore, their family relationship are cut off, and they are isolated and removed from families. After that day, I did not see Shuanglong return to the clinic; his mother never came back either.

I once asked Dr. Wang if Shuanglong could continue to take his anti-viral medication at the detox center. He replied, "The detox center also has its own clinic. Basically, we send the medications to the clinic monthly, and the clinic will take care of the rest of the issue." Dr. Wang stopped and sighed, "I don't know what to say about these patients. They are miserable but also detestable. I always have my sympathy toward them, they look so miserable when they got very sick; but I also hate them so much when they mess up like this. They just would not listen to you even if they are going to die. And they always lie to you. Every time I meet them, I ask them if they are still using drugs and warn them not to use it anymore, but they just lied to me. They hurt their own families so much that their families simply do not care if they are alive or dead at all. I really don't know what to do with them."

Yanping — Why Don't You Just Die?

There were about 20 female patients receiving anti-viral treatment at the clinic, Yanping was one of them. She was around 25 years old and married. According to her own narrative, she must have contracted AIDS from her ex-boyfriend whom she later found out was a drug user. Shortly after she married her current husband, she was diagnosed as HIV positive. Her husband was requested to take HIV testing too, right after she was confirmed as infected. Fortunately, her husband's test result turned out to be negative.

I had my first conversation with Yanping in a bar; sitting with us were two of my workmates who had been working in this adherence program for a year. They introduced me to Yanping and told her that they were leaving and I was going to take over their work in the program for the following several months. Yanping chose the place to meet us. She said that she preferred not to meet at the hospital because it always reminded her about her AIDS. Also, it was her birthday that day.

Yanping did not tell her parents about her AIDS status. "It was horrible. I didn't want them to know about it." She said. Out of shame, her husband also hid the situation from his own family, but he was extremely angry at her for hiding her past history, and he began mistreating her at home. Although Yanping started seeing her husband after she broke up with her ex-boyfriend, her husband still blamed her for unloyalty and called her a liar and "bitch". At the time I met Yanping, she and her husband still lived under the same roof in order to disguise the marriage that already fallen apart. But they were using separate spaces and utilities at home. Her husband tried to find every chance to pick on her and accuse her, "why don't you just die?"

I asked Yanping if she had thought about divorce, she said that she suggested that to her husband, but her husband refused to do so. "He was afraid that everybody would know the truth if we divorced. That would be a big shame to him and a deadly blow to our parents. He did not say so, but I could tell that was the reason he refused to divorce."

"Then what are you going to do? Do you have any plan for your future? Can you imagine living like that for the rest of your life?" I asked.

"I have no idea. I just plan one day at a time. Things have gone this far, lots of things are not for me to decide or make a choice."

I stopped, and then went on to talk about something else. After all, it was her birthday and I did not want to ruin it. Yanping was young and pretty. None would think of HIV/AIDS if they ran into her in the street. I looked around the bar. Many girls accompanied by their friends were enjoying the night: talking, laughing, and making fun of each other. I thought to myself that Yanping just looked like them and she could also have had the same happy life as they seemed to have. But her happy days were already gone.

In Dexin, there were many times when I was walking down the streets after work that I looked at people walking by slowly. The sky was bright and blue; the green leaves were flickering; the gentle breeze was warm. People, natives or tourists, all had smiles on their faces. But my mind was still full of what I heard from patients at the clinic; all kinds of pain and suffering were still resounding in my head. What a divided world! Sometimes I wondered what those patients would look like when they were walking on the same streets and how they would feel about what they saw around them. I also asked myself if these happy walkers knew that along with their happy lives another completely different life world was also going on at the same time; if they would care to know that; how would they respond if they got to know? There is no doubt that all people have their own unspeakable pain and suffering, and they do not necessarily put everything on their faces, but I believe that their suffering is hardly comparable to the ones I have observed and witnessed almost every day during my research period.

During my stay in Dexin, I had chances to meet Yanping several times. She came to the clinic once a month for medication refill. I asked Yanping if she had tried to have her husband come to the clinic for counseling, which was applied to help patients' families get to know what HIV/AIDS is about, teach them how to deal with the disease and protect themselves. The counseling program was planned to help families dissolve their misunderstanding about HIV/AIDS and also aimed to remove stigma from within families.

Yanping said, "I tried to talk to him about counseling. But he would not listen to me at all. In fact, he got angry with my suggestion. He said that my disease was my fault and it had nothing to do with him. He considered coming to the clinic for that kind of counseling a great shame and humiliation to him. He blamed me for trying to add to his shame by urging him to do the counseling." Her husband also called her a shameless person and shouted at her, "You have this shameless disease and you don't feel the shame. That is fine. How could you try to drag me into this? Why would I do that to humiliate myself?"

I told her that she could have asked Dr. Wang to help her and let Dr. Wang talk to her husband about the counseling. She replied with a bitter smile, "Actually, counseling was Dr. Wang's idea in the beginning. Otherwise, how could I have the courage to ask my husband to do the counseling? He was already extremely angry at me about my AIDS. When I told Dr. Wang that I failed to persuade my husband to come in for counseling, Dr. Wang tried to call him. My husband still refused to do so and he claimed that he has nothing to do with me."

Later I mentioned this to Dr. Wang. He told me, "The counseling program is a good idea. But if patients' families do not want to do it, there is nothing I can do about it. I cannot force them to do so." As I observed both in Beijing and Dexin, few family members would agree to come to the clinic for counseling. Volunteer counseling is a good program designed only if it works; apparently, it has never worked for most families. It only works when families still care about their patients, which I have not seen a lot, or when families misunderstand it as an obligatory program in which they have no choice but to participate. Help only works for those who want it. But what about those who do not feel they need help or simply refuse to be helped. In this sense, the volunteer counseling program is not as promising as was expected in dealing with stigma. Problematic is the basic assumption behind the counseling program and also the current anti-stigma campaign: (1) stigma associated with HIV/AIDS is caused by ignorance about HIV/AIDS; (2) possessing medical knowledge will eliminate stigma. In fact, the local moral meaning turns out to be a big obstruction that prevents people from accessing medical knowledge about HIV/AIDS. Compared to the question of how to make medical knowledge more accessible to patients' families and the general population, a more important issue that has to be considered is what happens if families and the general population do not care to know the medical knowledge or simply refuse to know it due to the local moral sense that it is shameful. According to a research conducted by Liu *et al.* (2006) in China, "HIV counseling reduced perceived worry but exerted little impact on HIV-related stigma and the intention (to disclose one's HIV/AIDS status)" (2006: 133).

The current education programs designed to fulfill the goal of the anti-stigma campaign seemed to have failed by applying scare techniques to frighten people away from deviant behaviors in order to prevent them from developing HIV/AIDS. The very failure has fostered and strengthened the local moral meaning inherent in stigma.

Wu *et al.* (2005) conducted a study on the acceptability of HIV/AIDS counseling and test among premarital couples in China and found that "acceptance of HIV test was disappointingly low" and one of the reasons "might have been the stigmatization associated with HIV test". "Specifically, a couple's relationship may be threatened if one of the partners is either identified as HIV positive or wants to be tested, revealing previous risky behavior" (2005: 12). As I have heard in my field research, many people believe that they don't have to worry about contracting HIV/AIDS because they have nothing to do with the disease. "I have never done those things. I am not that kind of person and I don't have those kinds of friends either. Why should I worry about it? Why should I know what kind of disease it is? Only those who did those things care to know this disease. If I have never done those things, why should I know about it? If someone wants to know, he must have done those things." "Those things" generally refer to using drugs and visiting prostitutes. Rather than ignorance, this response of being unwilling to know the relevant medical knowledge about HIV/AIDS is more a moral response to the perceived immoral things and persons associated with AIDS. It also indicates that stigma associated with HIV/AIDS is not caused by the disease itself; instead, it is a local moral judgment concerning what kind of persons "those people" are and what they have done that caused the disease.

Zhimei — Return My Pills; or I Am Going to Report You to the Police

Dr. Wang was well known for his long-term work in the field of HIV/AIDS. He was so strict in his work that most of the nurses and patients were afraid of him. Sometimes when nurses met some problematic patients whom they were unable to handle, they would report to Dr. Wang. Once Dr. Wang gets angry, the problem, it was thought, is soon going to be resolved. The clinic was managed like a big family with a patriarchal system, where Dr. Wang acted as the father, the head of nurses as the mother, and other young doctors and nurses as sons and daughters. Although it might not look professional enough, this system has been working just fine.[2]

I once asked Dr. Wang how he started working on HIV/AIDS. "It was a coincidence. I was not in the field at all, and I have never learnt about HIV/AIDS before that." About 10 years ago when he was working as the

---

[2]At this clinic, all doctors and nurses except Dr. Wang had never received professional trainings in treating HIV/AIDS or caring the HIV/AIDS patients. The other clinic's staff simply learned from Dr. Wang and worked under his instruction.

head of the dermatology department, he was once requested to participate in a joint diagnosis of two patients. "Those two patients had strange symptoms. We had several department heads working together, and we tried everything we could, but we still could not figure out the problem. We had no idea what kind of disease it was. Suddenly an article I had read from a medical journal came to my mind. It was about HIV/AIDS. But none of us had ever met HIV/AIDS cases before that. I suggested that we gave it a try, and the result confirmed my guess. That was how I found the first HIV/AIDS case at this hospital. After that, the hospital decided to let my department deal with HIV/AIDS cases. In the following few years I went to several medical schools in big cities, including Beijing, for professional training. You know, if I was going to work in this field, I definitely needed some professional training." Dr. Wang's experience is a lived example of the encounter between China and HIV/AIDS epidemic: the whole country was not ready at all when the epidemic hit. Medical professionals and the country both had to learn while dealing with the epidemic at the same time.

Dr. Wang told me about an accident that once happened to him several years ago, which almost caused him to be infected by HIV. "I was giving an HIV/AIDS patient surgery. The patient's blood was suddenly all over my face due to the malfunction of the surgical equipment. I was scared, but I tried to calm down to finish the surgery. After it was done, I immediately went to wash and clean my face for a long time. I was scared to death. I didn't tell my wife or parents. I decided to keep it to myself. I gave myself an HIV test. It was negative. But HIV/AIDS has a window-phase of three months, during which the virus cannot be tested. So I had to wait till the end of window-phase for another test. During that period, I spent each day as if it were a year. I just felt that each day was such a long time. I didn't tell anyone. I didn't dare to go home to face my wife, so every day I worked at my office till late at night to make sure that my wife was already asleep when I arrived home. It was such a long three-month. But fortunately the final test result turned out to be negative. Later when I told my wife about what had happened, she cried." I had heard stories similar to Dr. Wang's when I was working in Beijing. To some extent, these doctors had experienced the same feeling as their patients had. Although they didn't turn out to be HIV/AIDS patients in the end, more or less they were able to understand how HIV/AIDS patients felt and what they had been through. It is easy to criticize doctors when they are getting tough with patients, but it is unfair to blame them for having no sense at all about patients' suffering.

If I remember correctly, Zhimei was the only female drug user I met at Dr. Wang's clinic who contracted AIDS. She often showed up at the clinic with an attitude of never-minding anything. Sometimes when she came in, she appeared impatient to any question and did not want to say a single word; sometimes she came to the clinic right after she used drugs, she became extremely talkative, spoke to anybody she ran into, even felt free to sing in the clinic room.

Zhimei also participated in the adherence research project. Starting from the sixth month of the research, all patients were divided into two groups: Intervention group and control group. For the intervention group, when patients came in for medication refills, their electronic medication bottles were scanned and their adherence records were printed out. Doctors were supposed to examine the adherence records with patients together: Show patients when they missed the time for medication, find out why they missed, and help them figure out how to improve their medication adherence in the future. For the control group, records were also scanned and downloaded but not to show to anyone, neither medical staff nor patients themselves.

I soon found out that intervention often turned out to be a criticism session: When doctors or nurses had the adherence records in their hands and found the missing points, they turned to ask patients what happened and blamed patients for missing the time. They usually pointed at the dots (in the records) and asked, "What was going on? Why did you miss the time? I told you to always take medication on time." They were supposed to help patients find out the reason and help them improve their medication adherence, but in reality they began using the records as a weapon to blame patients. The intervention session became more like an interrogation. Sometimes they even asked me to show them the records that belonged to patients from the control group. Especially when they were not happy with some patients, they would do so. They wanted an excuse to blame and punish those patients. I always refused to do so because it was a protocol violation.

Zhimei was placed into the intervention group. When she came in for the seventh month, I scanned her bottle, downloaded the records, and then I found a problem. Patients were supposed to take medications twice a day, they usually do it in the morning and evening; hence there would be two dots a day on the records' sheet. The bottle could hold medications for a month. Therefore, when patients came in for refill, there would be about 60 dots on the records' sheet. But Zhimei's records showed only one dot; I checked the details of records and found out there were 59 dots in total, but all overlapped and looked like one dot. The precise time sheet showed that Zhimei opened the bottle 59 times during 2 min in the morning of the day she came to the clinic. Apparently, she fabricated her records, but she thought that the bottle could only memorize how many times she opened it. What she did not know was that the bottle also memorizes exactly what time it was opened, precisely in seconds. More problematic was that the records could not tell if she had really taken her medication or if she just opened the bottle in order to make it look like she had taken her medication. I said to myself, "Poor Zhimei!" I was worried what doctors and nurses were going to do to her.

When the nurses found out what Zhimei did, they became extremely angry and immediately began interrogating her. "What were you doing? What did you have in your mind? Just tell the truth, what did you do with your medications?" Zhimei seemed confused in the beginning because she didn't expect her trick would be exposed so soon. She hesitated and then started explaining. She insisted that she did take her medications and always took medications on time. While completely ignoring the records that nurses put in front of her, Zhimei repeated, "I did take my medications on time. I did what you told me to do, how could I know what happened to the bottle?"

The nurses would not let it go so easily. Zhimei was sitting on a chair while several nurses stood around her. A nurse asked, "You said that you took medications on time, but why do the records not say so? The records show that you only opened the bottle this morning; moreover, you kept opening and closing it 59 times. Could the bottle tell lies? I don't believe you. Take a look at the records, you'd better tell us the truth." Zhimei had nothing to say but kept saying that she did take medication on time.

Another nurse said to Zhimei, "We are doing this for your own good. Taking medication is your own business. Why are you so irresponsible to yourself? We will not lose anything if you don't take medication; we will not earn anything if you do. We just want you to be honest to yourself. If you do not want to take medications, then you should not have had this disease." The last sentence apparently irritated Zhimei. She stopped for a while and then became upset, "Yes, you are right. It is my own business. Then why do you care so much if I had my medications or not. It has nothing to do with you. Just leave me alone."

The Nurses were getting even angrier because they did not expect that Zhimei had the courage to fire back at them. In their opinion, patients were supposed to listen to medical staff all the time. They started shouting at Zhimei, "What did you mean by that? How could you say that? We are helping you. I cannot imagine what you just said to us." And then they threatened Zhimei, "Don't go anywhere, just sit here. Dr. Wang is coming in soon. We will see what he is going to do with you." Zhimei became nervous and said, "I have to go. I have some issues to take care of today." The nurses ignored her and turned to me, "Please don't give her money until Dr. Wang comes in. He has to know this. We cannot handle it." Zhimei already stood up and tried to leave; once she heard nurses say so, she stopped. Apparently 150 yuan each month means a lot for her; she would not leave until she got the money. I felt that I was trapped in a dilemma; first, I did not like the nurses to accuse Zhimei in this way; secondly, I did not want to refuse the nurses' request, which would make them lose face in front of patients. Since the intervention was supposed to be done by medical staff, I had to wait for Dr. Wang to see if he could do something about this situation.

While we were waiting for Dr. Wang, several other patients came in for medication refill. Zhimei became vexed and kept asking what time Dr. Wang was coming in. The nurses ignored her question, ordered her to wait outside the office and make some room for other patients. After half an hour, Dr. Wang showed up at the clinic. When he heard the report from several nurses and read Zhimei's records, he slapped the sheets at his desk and started shouting at Zhimei, "What is wrong with you? Are you out of your mind?"

Zhimei was standing in front of his desk, and she still tried to explain, "Dr. Wang, I did take my medications. I told the truth. I don't know what was going on with the bottle."

"You just keep lying, do you? Do you think that I am so stupid that I believe that? Cut the crap!"

Zhimei became silent while looking down at the floor.

"I know you people very well. Just don't lie to me, don't try to fool me. You are still using drugs, aren't you?"

"No, I am not."

"Great! I am going to give you a drug testing right now. You just keep lying." Dr. Wang rushed into another clinic room and came back with a drug test package. He slapped the package on his desk and told Zhimei to go to the bathroom and get her urine tested. "If your test turns out to be positive, I am going to call the detox center right away and ask them to take you in."

Zhimei immediately surrendered and started crying. She stayed where she was standing and did not move.

Dr. Wang said with a victorious facial expression, "Scared? You thought I could not deal with you, didn't you? You just won't cry until you see a coffin. (Extremely stubborn, never give up until the last minute) What did you do with my pills? Just be honest!"

Zhimei sobbed, "I did not take it. I am sorry. I made a mistake and I admit it now. Please forgive me."

"Why didn't you take the pills?"

"I have a boyfriend right now. I didn't tell him that I have this disease. And I am afraid that he was going to find out the truth if he saw me taking these pills. The bottle looks so strange and it attracts a lot of attention."

A nurse stepped in and said, "You could have taken your pills at a private place such as bathroom when your boyfriend was not around. I know many patients are doing so. You could have figured out a way to do it. It is not a big problem at all."

"You don't understand. It is not that simple. The bottle just scared the hell out of me. It made me nervous all the time."

Dr. Wang did not care about her story, and went on to interrogate Zhimei. "What did you do with the pills? Don't tell me that you threw all those pills away."

Zhimei immediately denied it and said, "No, no, I did not. I just took them out of the bottle and put them in some place at home."

"Don't lie to me. The pills are all provided by the government for free. Do you have any idea how much it costs to the government? Do you have any idea how many patients do not have access to these pills and have to wait for death? I am telling you, if you throw those pills away, you are committing a crime. I have the right to report you to the police and let them arrest you. It is a crime." Dr. Wang was just trying to scare Zhimei; throwing pills was not a crime in a legal sense. But he was definitely able to send Zhimei to the detox center and make her suffer.

Dr. Wang continued, "Where did you put those pills? Listen, bring me back my pills tomorrow; otherwise I am going to report you to the police." And then he said to me, "Don't give her money until she comes back with those pills." I had to do as Dr. Wang requested.

After the nurses refilled Zhimei's medication bottle, she left; she did not show up the next day. In fact, she never showed up with those pills. Later Dr. Wang said to me, "I knew that she already threw those pills away. How could she bring them back? A patient like her really gives me a headache. What can I do? Just let it go. They just keep lying to you."

The good thing was that after the criticism session Zhimei's adherence records showed that she was getting on track to take her medication. I gave her money back when she visited the clinic in the following month. That was what I could do.

After this incident, I started paying attention to how patients feel about using their electronic bottle. I did not expect that the bottle became a trouble to patients who were using it. I also found out that the bottle could be cheated and played with, though Zhimei was not successful in doing so. In fact, I found a successful example. I was not sure how many patients were cheating on the bottle; but at least I knew one; a patient admitted it to me. He was doing paoche business, driving a bus for tourists. He said that he had no way to always take medication on time because he was working almost 24 hours a day. But he was smart enough to figure out a way that his bottle records always show that he had never missed his medication time. When he went back home after the bottle was refilled at the clinic, he took all pills out of the electronic bottle and put them in another bottle, and then he gave the empty electronic bottle to his son and asked him to open it on time twice a day. In doing so, he could take pills anytime when he was free; while the empty electronic bottle could still memorize the time when it was opened, thought it meant nothing.

I promised the patient not to tell anyone at the clinic about his cheating on the bottle. But I still warned him to do his best to take medications on time. He said, "Mei banfa (I have no choice). Doctors asked me to join this research, how could I say no to them? In addition, I can earn 150 yuan each month. It is not a big money, but it's better than nothing. I know you are a good person and trying to help us. I did not mean to cheat on you, but I have no choice. Anyway I will try my best." I had enough reason to believe that he was not the only one who figured out a way to cheat.

Although Dr. Wang's way of dealing with patients seemed to have been very successful and effective in his clinic, his method is an example of stigmatization within medical institution. Criticism, frightening patients, humiliation, and punishment are the usual methods applied by medical professionals in their routine working with drug users and HIV/AIDS patients. They use these methods to get patients on medication and to do what they think is right. They believe that they are doing right things for patients' own good. At the clinic, patients' rights of being a person with subjectivity and agency were denied and ignored. Patients were treated as children who have no sense of what really matters for themselves. What medical professionals care about are symptoms, medications, and test results rather than patients' daily lives and personal suffering. For drug users who contracted HIV/AIDS, medical professionals treat them as non-persons and blame them as criminals who have committed crimes against society and their own families, and also as liars who have never spoken truth to anyone.

Yali — You Have No Sense of Shame

Using an electronic bottler became a problem for patients like Zhimei: if they took pills on time, they were afraid that their AIDS status would be exposed; if they did, they were going to be criticized by the clinic's staff. However, for some patients, the bottle came to be a symbol of stigma rather than a problem in their daily lives.

Yali was living in a distant village. Several years before, her husband died from either using drugs or AIDS, nobody knows for sure. After her husband died, Yali tested HIV positive. She was living with her daughter and her husband's parents at the time. A nurse told me that Yali cried a lot when she came to the clinic during the first several months, but she felt better recently.

When I met Yali for the first time, she was accompanied by her mother-in-law. After she sat down, her mother-in-law went to another clinic room, and I began asking Yali the usual questions. She looked at me and started crying without saying a single word. I was confused because she looked just fine when she came in and I did not say anything wrong. Having heard her cry, a nurse and her mother-in-law came in to comfort her. The nurse explained to me that Yali did not speak Mandarin. I did not know that. Because most of the patients I met at the clinic all spoke Mandarin, I just assumed that she spoke Mandarin too. While they were communicating in the Bai language, I could sense that Yali cried not because she could not understand Mandarin. I asked the nurse what happened. She would not tell me the truth. But I came to realize that Yali misunderstood me and thought I said something bad to her. I could sense it from her facial expression. I started apologizing; I told her that I did not know that she did not speak Mandarin and whatever she heard from me was not what I meant to say. I asked the nurse to translate my words to Yali. Yali would not stop and kept crying, while her mother-in-law and the nurse were trying to explain to her and comfort her.

I passed a napkin to Yali, which she would not take it. Her mother-in-law did so for her. I had to say sorry again and explained again that I did not mean to hurt her feeling. I was sitting in front of her and could not figure out what to do. I had been learning the Bai language from a friend, a doctor at the clinic; but the Bai language has many local dialects. I could not understand even a single word Yali spoke.

Yali stopped crying but kept sobbing silently. And then she said something to me. I asked the nurse what she said.

"She does not want to use the electronic bottle anymore."

"Ok, no problem. It is up to you, really. If you do not want to use it, then do not use it. Nobody is going to force you to use it." I was so eager to make her feel better that I agreed to her request without any hesitation. And then I asked why.

After the nurse, Yali, and her mother-in-law communicated in the Bai language for a while, I got the translation and also the answer from the nurse. Yali had been worried about the bottle. It looked strange (it had a yellow body with a big white cap, and a code number was attached to the body); and it would beep whenever it was opened or closed. The bottle made Yali nervous all the time. She had been taking care of this bottle as a secret and always tried to make sure that none outside her family would find out. But there is no secret in a village no matter how deeply you hide it. When some villagers found out that she was using the strange bottle, they kept asking her what it was. Every time when she was asked, she had to make up an excuse to disguise the truth. It became a great pressure on her and made her extremely stressed. Every time when she was using the bottle or when she was asked about it, she was reminded that she had AIDS.

Yali also considered the bottle a treasure that she had received from the clinic and she had the obligation to protect the bottle and keep it intact. Yali once visited a relative and spent a few days at the relative's place. When she went home after the visit, she found out that she left the bottle at her relative's home. She was so nervous that she had to go back to her relative's place the same night to take back her bottle. She was afraid that her relative would find out her secret; she was also worried that she could lose her bottle or have it damaged.

When Yali finally found the bottle at her relative's place, her relatives seemed both confused and curious. They did not understand why such a bottle was so important that Yali had to get it back even at late night. They asked her about it. Yali had to tell her relative that it was just medication for her liver. The relatives seemed uncomfortable with Yali's coming back for the bottle late at night; they teased her by saying, "You don't have to worry about that. If it is left at our place, it is going to be safe. Nobody in our family will take it from you. You will not lose it. It is just a pill bottle. We do not want it and we will send it back to you later. You don't have to come over to get it back at night." Yali felt she was humiliated and cried on her way back home. "It was shame the bottle brought to me." Yali said.

Yali had a daughter who was in a local elementary school. After her husband died, her daughter's school fee had been waived as a subsidy to the family. Soon after the school found out that the girl's father might have died from using drugs or from AIDS, and there were also rumors in the village that the girl's mother might also have contracted AIDS, they decided to cancel the subsidy and ask Yali to pay for her daughter's school fee. Yali became angry with the school's decision. "No matter what the kid's parents have done, it has nothing to do with the kid." Yali said. She went to her daughter's school and questioned the school's principle. She was told that it was determined by local policy and the school could do nothing about it. When she asked for the government document that was said to state the policy, the principle would not show her any document but kept saying it was government policy. When Yali expressed her anger and disappointment with the school's decision, the principle became mad at her and warned her to leave: "You know what your husband has done, and you are also very clear about your own situation. I cannot imagine such a person like you still has the courage to come here and argue with me. Go home; don't lose your own face even further! I did not ask your daughter to leave my school, so I think I am kind enough. You should thank me. You have no sense of shame at all."

Yali started crying aloud when she was telling this story. Given the fact that she could do nothing to change the way other people had been treating her and her family, it was understandable that she turned her anger to the bottle she was using. She said, "It was all about this bottle. I hate it. I do not want to use it anymore. It is such a shame." I tried to comfort her, "It is alright. If you do not want to use it, then do not use it. It is your call. I have no problem with that." Yali's mother appeared worried that Yali might irritate me by insisting not to use the bottle; she tried to explain, "She did not mean it. She just had a hard time. She will be fine."

I passed another napkin to Yali; she took it this time. I repeated that she does not have to use the bottle and she can quit the research anytime she wants. She did not say yes or no, but kept sobbing.

When Yali was back to her normal mood, she told me that her bottle had a problem: sometimes it would not beep when it was opened or closed. I told her that the battery might be down, and then I replaced her bottle. I asked her again and wanted to make sure if she really wanted to continue using the bottle. She nodded. I had nothing to say, but I was not sure if I did a right thing by letting her keep the bottle. "Maybe she was just stressed and needed a moment," I said to myself.

After Yali left with her mother-in-law, a nurse said to me, "If you let her quit the program, she won't get 150 yuan each month. That money can be a big help to her family since her husband already died and she does not have a job now."

The following month Yali showed up in high spirit at the clinic. I felt relaxed and happy for her. She was good at making hand-made embroidery, which was called shizi xiu (literally cross embroidery) in local words, a very popular needlework among Bai women. Yali brought in her needlework to the clinic and shared with us. Several nurses were chasing her around, asking her to teach them how to do it. Watching them communicating about embroidery, I comforted myself that I might have done the right thing by keeping her in this program.

Weiqiang — We Don't Care if He Is Alive or Dead

Weiqiang was a patient I will never forget. In fact, I only had one talk with him, but two days after the talk I heard about his death. For quite a while I had been thinking that his death had some kind of relation with our conversation.

Weiqiang was about 43 years old, short and a little bald. He was one of the quietest patients I had met at the clinic. It was maybe his age, older than most of patients, that made him not that social among the patients' group. He often came in and left alone, occasionally with another patient, Dawei, who I believe was his only friend. When he came in for medicine refill, he would never speak to anyone at first; he just answered questions in a few words.

One day when I came to the clinic, I found out that Weiqiang was hospitalized. A nurse told me that the staff on duty last night received a call from Dawei, Weiqiang's only friend, saying that Weiqiang was in a critical condition. The staff reported it to Dr. Wang, and then Dr. Wang drove to Weiqiang's place and brought him back to the clinic. Weiqiang was hospitalized that night. I was confused why it was not his family but Dawei who made that call for help. Dr. Wang told me that Weiqiang had been kicked out of his family several years before after he was found HIV positive, and after that he had been living alone. Only his friend, Dawei, occasionally went over to check on his condition.

Weiqiang had been lying in a ward bed for several days, and then he seemed to be getting better. Sometimes I saw him sitting outside the ward and enjoying the sunshine. He was always quiet, sitting there without a word or any facial expression. He could even maintain the same posture for the whole afternoon. Sometimes when I met him at the hospital's small dining room, he did not speak a word but gave me a smile.

Dr. Wang complained to me about Weiqiang's family. "I called his family several times, asking them if they could send somebody over to take care of Weiqiang, but they refused to do so. They claimed that Weiqiang has nothing to do with them and they had not minded Weiqiang's business for a long time." Dr. Wang mimicked Weiqiang's family on the phone, "We do not care if he's alive or dead. It is not our business." Then Dr. Wang started shaking his head, "I don't know what to say about this kind of family. We are trying hard to save these patients' lives, but their families already gave up on them." Dr. Wang said that he once asked Weiqiang's family at least to pay for the hospitalization fee, though they did not want to come over to take care of him. But his family insisted that they were not going to pay any fee for Weiqiang and they did not care who was going to pay.

"Then what are you going to do with the bills?" I asked.

"Mei banfa. (I have no choice) Fortunately we have some extra funding; I think I have to use that money to pay for it." Dr. Wang kept shaking his head, "What else can I do?"

I was quite busy that week. Many patients came in for medication refills and program interviews. When I finally found a chance to talk to Weiqiang, it was a Friday; he was going home soon that day. I decided to talk to him before he left. It was almost 5 in the afternoon. All of the clinic's staff left and the ward area was empty; Weiqiang was the only one who was hospitalized at the time.

I asked Weiqiang questions concerning his history of using drugs. He always answered in short sentences or several words in an unbelievably calm manner. I passed a cigarette to him and tried to make the talk informal and personal. He looked at me for a second, smiled and then took it over. I lit the cigarette for him; his fingers were shaking. His eyes looked brighter.

"Are you married?"

"No."

"Ever had a girl friend?"

"Ah! Never had one." Weiqiang shook his head with a smile on his face, and then looked up at the ceiling. "Look at me, is anyone willing to be with me?"

"What about your family? Are you still living with them?"

"No, I moved out."

"So you are living by yourself now?"

"Yes."

"Was it your idea or your family asked you to leave?"

Weiqiang seemed uncomfortable with this question. He turned around not to look at me, "Actually, it is good for me to move out. It is good for both my family and me. If I move out, my family will not be troubled anymore."

"What kind of trouble?"

"This disease is dangerous. And also many people were talking about my family because of my disease."

Weiqiang did not answer my question whether or not he was asked by his family to leave. He would not admit it because of the shame attached to being abandoned by his own family.

"Where are you living now?"

"A separate place. Not far from my family."

"Has you family ever come to see you at your place?"

"Not really. Sometimes I went back to see them."

"How do you eat? Do you make food for yourself?"

"No. I go back to eat with my parents."

"For every meal?"

"No, just sometimes. Several times a week."

"Then what do you do for every day?"

Weiqiang smiled, "There is nothing I can do. Just stay at my place, sometimes I go out with friends."

"Then what were you doing with your friends?"

"Nothing, just for fun. Killing some time."

Weiqian once had a job at a local factory. He was found hiding drugs at his dormitory, and then he was fired. The factory also informed his parents about his using drugs and asked them to bring their son back home. With such a stain, he could never find a job after that. For drug users like Weiqiang, their life histories seemed almost blank: no job, no love, and no family life. Their normal life tracks had been cut off since they were caught using drugs. Since that day, the whole world had completely changed for them; they started living with criticism, accusation, avoidance, refusal, isolation, and discrimination.

Weiqiang was sitting in front of me; I did not have a clue about what he had in his mind. I asked questions, he answered; when I stopped, he stopped talking too. I went on to ask if he had any question about medications and treatment or if he had any difficulty in taking medications on time. He said no to all of my questions. I asked him if he felt better after staying at the hospital for a week. He said, "Yes, much better."

I had to stop; it was a short talk but I thought that he might talk more when we got more familiar with each other in the future. "It is a good beginning. We still have time and we can talk later." I said to myself. So I ended the conversation.

Slowly, Weiqiang put on his coat, packed his stuff that he had used during his hospitalization with a used plastic bag, and then left. While he was doing so, I was watching him. Before he left, he looked back at me and gave me a smile. I saw a bizarre color in his eyes; but soon it skipped out of my mind.

On Monday morning, when I walked into the clinic, Dr. Wang said, "Weiqiang died on Friday night." I was shocked. Although AIDS is well known as a deadly disease, it was the first time a patient who I knew died during my field research; moreover, I might have been the last person to whom Weiqiang ever talked. Soon Weiqiang's appearance and words from our last conversation came to my mind; I started thinking that there was some kind of connection between the conversation and his death. I also began replaying our last talk, trying to find out if I had said or did something wrong to Weiqiang.

Dr. Wang said, "Weiqiang might have died of epilepsy. I guess that his epilepsy broke out that night and nobody was there to help him because he was living alone. Then he just died that way. If he had been living with his family, he could have been saved." Dr. Wang sighed and went on to say, "That night Dawei went to Weiqiang's place and Weiqiang didn't answer the door. He thought Weiqiang was not home, and then he went to Weiqiang's family's place to find him. It turned out that Weiqiang was not with his family either. Dawei had a bad feeling and went back to Weiqiang's place. He broke in and found Weiqiang already dead in bed."

Although Dr. Wang said that Weiqiang died of epilepsy, I could not stop thinking that I was somehow involved in his death. It made me feel guilty. Later when Dawei came to the clinic, I talked about Weiqiang's death with him. He said, "His family did not care about him at all. If they did not kick Weiqiang out of family, he would not have died like that. You know what? When I found Weiqiang dead, and I ran over to let his family know about this, they even told me that they were not going to do anything about it. They did not even go to Weiqiang's place to take a look at him. They hoped that he would have died much earlier. I cannot believe there was such a kind of family, so cruel and inhuman."

That is what I know about Weiqiang. The conversation I had with him was the shortest of those I had with the patients at the clinic; but it was the one that impressed me most and came to my mind most frequently. Later I recalled the conversation from time to time, but I could hardly remember more than what I wrote above. His story was another example of family stigmatization: an HIV/AIDS patient was abandoned by his families. I believe that it is not a rare case. However, thinking so has never made me feel better because an HIV/AIDS patient's death has never been so close to me. I felt that I seemed to have witnessed his death; in fact, I was not there at all. I was merely one of those who heard about his death.

Summary

In this chapter, I focus on stigma related to HIV/AIDS among drug users who contract HIV/AIDS through sharing needles. Compared to HIV/AIDS patients I met in Beijing, the patients I interviewed in Dexin apparently were in poor family and financial situation. Most of them quit school early in the past and had no job; they divorced or never married. For these patients, stigma related to HIV/AIDS is associated with that related to drug abuse. They could hardly differentiate one from another.

Most of these patients had a long history of experience of being isolated and discriminated against for using drugs both in society and in the family. In general, drug users are already socially isolated and excluded before they are found to have contracted HIV/AIDS. No work unit would hire them. They are left uncared for or abandoned by their families. Shuanglong and Weiqiang's cases indicate that drug users are considered criminals who commit serious crimes to their own families and have no sense of family responsibility. Hence, for patients like Shuanglong, stigma related to HIV/AIDS added nothing new to their lives, which were already in the worst situation; it was just the continuum and extension of the worst situation.

The responses of the local government and other institutions to drug abuse strengthened the stigma related to drug abuse. As Dawei's story shows, the local detox center informed the drug users' parents' work units and used humiliation to punish not only the drug users but also their families. Shame and humiliation are also used by the local government as a legitimate way to mobilize anti-drugs war in society.

For patients like Yanping who was not a drug users but a victim of drug user, she contracted AIDS from her ex-boyfriend who was a drug user. Her story shows how an innocent victim was stigmatized and mistreated in the family. She might be innocent in the eyes of society, but definitely not in the eyes of her husband. She was blamed for being unloyalty and treated as an immoral woman in the family. Her HIV/AIDS status was considered treachery and shame to the family.

Zhimei's case demonstrates that stigmatization against HIV/AIDS patients also exists among the medical professionals. The way Zhimei was treated in the clinic shows how medical professionals feel about drug users and HIV/AIDS patients behind their routine medical practices. Doctors and nurses considered Zhimei a liar because of her drug abuse. They regarded governmental AIDS policy — free medication for HIV/AIDS patients — as a favor granted by the state, the local government, the hospital, the clinic, and certainly including themselves to HIV/AIDS patients. Such a view makes medical professionals to believe that they have the privilege to criticize, blame and threaten Zhimei when they found out that she did not take medication as was expected. In their opinion, Zhimei did not show her respect to the favor; moreover, being a non-person, she simply did not deserve the favor.

Chapter Five

A comparative perspective

Stigma Associated with Mental Illness Versus HIV/AIDS

I have presented my ethnography on stigma related to mental illness and HIV/AIDS respectively in the previous chapters. A comparative study, specifically focusing on the similarities and differences between the stigma related to the two illnesses, is needed to look further into the question of stigma *per se*. Through such a comparison, this chapter aims to explore, in the local context of China, how perceived cause and consequence of mental illness and HIV/AIDS as well as their lived experiences craft particular patterns or types of stigma. That is to say, I seek to understand via this comparison what stigma is about, why it matters so much, and what can be done about it.

After I started my field research, I often had to explain to my friends why I worked on both mental illness and HIV/AIDS; they often ignored my explanation and quibbled that I was only interested in those who had both mental illness and HIV/AIDS. It was a joke and in the beginning it seemed impossible to find such subjects who have both illnesses. Later when I began conducting research on HIV/AIDS, I soon found that among such patients, mental illness, especially depression, was not rare at all. Based on a study conducted in China, Jin *et al.* (2006) found high rates of depression (79%) and suicidal thoughts (18%) among the HIV/AIDS patients; despite the high rates, few (9%) had sought mental health assistance. (2006: 269) Nonetheless, an HIV/AIDS patient who suffers depression mostly from HIV/AIDS is not exactly the kind of subject my friends talked about, someone who was supposed to have independently contracted mental illness and HIV/AIDS. I didn't intend to specifically interview such a subject, but as it happened I did meet such a person when I was doing research at the AIDS Care Center in Beijing.

Tianyu — He Is a Retarded Shenjingbing

Mrs. Ding, the director of the AIDS Care Center, mentioned Tianyu to me during my first week at the Center. She spoke of Tianyu as a problematic AIDS patient who often lied; she wanted me to talk with him to see if there was anything she could do to help him. I said, no problem; upon hearing this, Zhanshan made a face at me and then burst into laughter. I was confused and asked him why; he just would not answer my question and kept saying, "You will see."

It was a Friday. When I walked into the Center in the morning, Mrs. Ding was talking with several patients. She introduced me to Tianyu, who was maybe two or three years older than me, tall and a little chubby. Mrs. Ding asked Tianyu to feel free to talk with me. Tianyu immediately moved his chair over and sat beside me. With a shiny smile on his face, he started talking. He was really talkative.

"It is good to have you here," he said.

"I also like to work with you guys." I replied.

"I don't like the other patients," he went on.

"Why?"

"They do not like to talk with me," Tianyu complained.

As I could remember, all the patients I met at the Center treated each other as brothers and sisters. They came together to the Center and shared with each other what was going on most recently in their lives. They liked to keep each other company. Hence, when I heard this statement from Tianyu, I was surprised. During our talk, nobody came up to speak to Tianyu, which was not normal at the Center. Usually, no matter whom I was talking with, others would come over from time to time just to make fun or join the conversation. They were all friends; they did not consider it rude to cut in to other people's conversation. Moreover, they already knew each other very well. They knew each other's families, personal lives and how they contracted AIDS. Basically, there was no secret among this patient group; they had nothing to hide from each other. They never felt that they need a space to hold a private conversation. However, when I was talking with Tianyu, all the other patients tried to avoid or ignore him.

Tianyu seemed to enjoy his conversation with me, and he tried to keep his voice low all the time as if we were having a very private chat. I did not feel comfortable with this, because I already had gotten used to speaking a little louder in the same way as those patients spoke to each other at the Center. At times, Tianyu touched my knee, trying to make us feel close to each other. In the Chinese context, social distance is not as far as defined in West society; touching somebody's arms, shoulders, or back is often used in interpersonal interactions. However, to touch someone is not just a friendly gesture; instead, it is more the embodiment of guanxi (interpersonal relationships), indicating a good and close guanxi. Whether or not you touch someone depends on existing guanxi: it is also based on the common intention and agreement from both parties to the interaction to get closer and make guanxi deeper. In general, strangers are not supposed to touch each other at all; otherwise, it will be considered not only rude but also stupid because it shows that the person has no sense of guanxi. Such a person is generally teased and blamed for bu dong shi (not knowing about the affair), meaning that a person does not understand the affair of guanxi, does not know how to act within the existing interpersonal relationship, and is interacting inappropriately with others.

I came to understand Zhanshan's facial gesture and what Tianyu meant when he complained that the other patients did not like to talk with him. While I was talking with Tianyu, Zhanshan made another face at me and then left the room. I learned from Tianyu about his family and how he had contracted AIDS. Tianyu was born into a family in Beijing. He had a married older sister and a twin brother. Tianyu quit school when he was in his second year of senior high school, and then joined the army to serve in Shanxi Province. In 1996, after four years he was dismissed from the army, and he returned to Bejing to find a job. He wanted to work in the railway system, which he had dreamed about for a long time, but he could not find such a job. Instead, he had to work on the security staff in a work unit, where he was fired for no reason.

Tianyu believed that he contracted AIDS through homosexual intercourse and admitted that he was a gay. But he clarified that he was not born a gay; instead he attributed his gay identity to gay men's sexual seduction. He told me that he was kidnapped and then raped by a gay man when he was 16 years old. And then he went on to describe how he had been seduced by this and other gay man.

"It was their fault; they made me a gay." Tianyu complained.

"How did you meet them?" I asked.

"I did not know them; they found me." Tianyu said with an angry expression on his face.

Tianyu narrated this and other events to me. He even described how he was instructed to do oral sex for gay men, in detail. I did not ask about it, nor did I mean to get to know about it, especially in detail. Tianyu mentioned it himself and started talking about it in endless detail. I was not feeling comfortable with this turn in the conversation and turned silent. Tianyu seemed to be unable to recognize my reticence to get into this topic and kept talking about it; moreover, he seemed to have no sense at all how embarrassing it was to talk about this issue with a person he had just met. Given the great shame of talking about sex in traditional Chinese culture, even though sex jokes have become increasingly common and popular in present China, Chinese people don't talk about sex in public, especially in such a formal or serious way in front of strangers. Most of the AIDS patients I met at the AIDS Care Center were gay men; most of them were able to talk with me at ease when we became familiar with each other. However, none of them ever felt easy enough to get into this topic in such detail when they were talking with me. To be honest, I was shocked. It was absolutely unexpected. I immediately had the thought, which I believe would come to any Chinese person's mind if he or she were in my situation: Tianyu must have had some problem with his brain because he had no sense at all about what to say or not to say in front of a specific person at a particular moment under certain circumstance. I also came to realize what Zhanshan was hinting at about Tianyu.

I did not interrupted Tianyu but waited for some moments to change the topic. I turned to ask how he found out about his AIDS. Eventually he changed the topic. In 2000, Tianyu had a persistent high fever, which lasted several months. At first, he tested HIV positive at another hospital, and then his AIDS status was confirmed at the hospital where the AIDS Care Center was located. Tianyu sighed, "It was all about bad luck. I always run into troubles. I have been so unlucky." I asked him how his family responded to his AIDS status; he immediately complained about his twin brother. Tianyu described his brother as an enemy.

"After I tested HIV positive, my brother started qishi (discriminate against) me." It was the first time I heard a patient using the term qishi to describe how he was mistreated by his family members. Although the patients I had met would talk about how they were mistreated by their family members and others outside their families, most of the time they preferred not to use the term qishi directly. They would prefer to describe the real situation that happened in daily life in detail, rather than use the term qishi.

"My brother began calling me aizibing (AIDS) at home and even in public. He said that I should die as soon as possible. He even told everybody that I had AIDS." Tianyu complained. That his brother became angry with him and even cursed him, saying he should die, I found common among the families with an AIDS member. But what I could not understand was why Tianyu's brother spoke of his AIDS in public and even told others about it. It is just not a normal family response to AIDS. As I observed from my research, all families tended to hide the AIDS status from others outside the family; sometimes they even concealed it from the other family members in order to hide the shame and protect the family from the stigma. Upon hearing Tianyu's complaint, his brother's destructive behavior did not make any sense to me. I started to have the thought that Tianyu's brother might also have a mental disorder. Later my guess was confirmed by Mrs. Ding, Zhanshan and the other patients.

Tianyu went on, "I am like a slave at home. I have to do all the housework and even cook for my brother. But I am starving all the time."

"What about your parents? Are you two living with your parents?" I asked.

"No, we are not living together. They are living in Shunyi (a district north of Beijing)."

I wanted to ask why their parents left him and his brother and moved to a separate place, but Tianyu apparently had not finished complaining, "Yesterday he waved a kitchen knife toward me and chased me around.

He threatened to kill me." I was shocked again. I did not know what to say and looked toward Mrs. Ding. She slightly shook her head to me while she was smiling. I recalled that she once reminded me that Tianyu often lied.

Tianyu kept talking all that morning. Before when I interviewed patients, I often had to make patients talk with me, stimulate them to talk more and change the topics from time to time to keep the conversation running; but Tianyu was completely another type of patient who would talk about everything with you, even if you did not ask any question. Moreover, what bothered me most was that Tianyu kept staring at me all the time and followed me everywhere I went.

At noon that day, I was surprised to find that I felt relieved; it was the first time in my field work that I felt the need to have a break from the conversation with an informant. Honestly, I was almost exhausted. We had lunch together with Mrs. Ding, Zhanshan and several other patients at the Center. During the lunch time, Tianyu sat beside me and still peeked at me from time to time while he was eating. After the lunch, I felt ready to call off the interview and take that afternoon off. Although we stopped, Tianyu kept staring at me no matter what I was doing and followed me no matter where I went. Even when I went to the bathroom, he still tried to follow me; fortunately he was stopped by Zhanshan. Tianyu just would not leave me alone. I did not feel it right to ask him to stop doing that; moreover, I suspected that he would not listen to me. Soon, Tianyu and I exchanged our roles in the interview; he began asking questions and I came to be the one to answer. Tianyu asked me where my hometown was, where I had been studying, even where I bought my clothes. Sometimes I answered; other times I simply ignored his questions. During our intermittent conversation, Tianyu asked me for my cell phone number; I hesitated at first and then gave it to him. I believed that I would have refused to do so if I was not doing this research.

At five in the afternoon, we left the Center and went home. When Tianyu found out that we were going in the same direction, he was happy; I felt exactly the opposite. When we finally got on a bus, we found that there was no spare seat. We had to stand side by side. Tianyu stared at me and said that I had been nice to him. I felt a little sorry for him.

"You are different from the other volunteers I met before." Tianyu said with a gentle smile on his face.

"Why is that?"

"You are nice. Those volunteers I met before would not talk much with me. Sometimes they were very hostile to me and even refused to talk with me." Tianyu complained that some volunteers he met before even told the other patients what they heard from him, "They are supposed to help us keep the secret. How could they tell others what I told them about myself?" My guess was that those volunteers and the other patients very likely made fun of him when he was not present. Later I found that many patients simply avoided and ignored Tianyu. In general, they would not speak a single word to him; when they did, they were teasing him. Most of the time, Tianyu could not figure out what others really meant; other times he could sense it.

It was a hot day and the bus was crowded. Tianyu touched my arm and expressed his concern about me, "You are sweating." I had no idea how to respond to that and said nothing. Tianyu turned to complain again about his brother. He repeated that his brother discriminated against him and told everybody about his AIDS status. He spoke of AIDS aloud while we were surrounded by the other bus riders. A middle-aged woman looked back at us. I was not sure if she overheard the term — AIDS. Tianyu seemed not to notice or mind at all. The HIV/AIDS patients usually avoid speaking of AIDS in public for fear that their AIDS status may be disclosed; they are also very sensitive when others mention the word in front of them in public. But Tianyu seemed to have no such sense: Either he did not sense the risk under such circumstance, or he simply did not have the sense of risk at all. I felt a little embarrassed, but it was not over yet. Tianyu started asking how I felt about the AIDS patients, how I felt about the other patients at the Center and how I felt about him. I kept my voice down, worrying that others could have heard us. I hinted to him not to talk about this in public; he just did not get it.

"How do you feel about me? Do you think I am danchun (innocent, ingenuous, simple-minded, and lack of knowledge of evil)?" I came to sense what he really meant to ask.

"You guys are all nice." I replied.

"Would you like to jiaowang with me?" Jiaowang means making friends in Chinese, which is usually applied to love relationship. To start jiaowang means to start a love relationship. If it was in another situation,

I would explain to him; but under such circumstance, on a bus with many people around us, I just wanted to end that topic as soon as possible. I decided to pretend that I did not understand what he really meant. Hence, I replied, "I like to make friends with all of you." Hearing my answer, Tianyu did not say a single word but smiled at me. Apparently, he did not sense the difference between his question and my answer, or he just took my answer the way he liked.

After several stops, Tianyu had to transfer to another bus and headed to his own place. I felt so relieved when he got off the bus; a feeling I had never experienced before during my field research. That night, Tianyu called me, asking me if I would go to the Center the next Monday and saying that he would like to meet me there. After I hung up the phone, I could not help recalling how Tianyu had acted and what he had said during that day. Although my intuition told me that Tianyu had mental illness, I had another thought that he might just be so lonely that he was eager to find a friend, find someone to talk to, and find someone who would at least listen to him, given the fact that he was marked and isolated even within the patient group.

I had to admit that Tianyu really made me feel annoyed and harassed. It was the first time I felt that way with my patient informants during my field research. To be honest, after I started this research, I met and made close contact with many people, such as the mentally ill, HIV/AIDS patients, gay men, sex workers, and drug users, whom I had never met in person before in my life. I learned about a variety of life styles, ideas and beliefs which are completely different from what I had been familiar with; I also made friends with most of them, some of them became my closest friends. Before I began this research, I was a little worried if I would be able to get along with individuals from these groups or conduct my research smoothly. However, once it started, I found it not as difficult as I expected. The contact and daily interaction I made with these patients seemed not that different from the ones I had with my other friends. Despite the fact that they were suffering from some painful or deadly diseases, these patients were just like other people: They also had normal emotions and concerns; they managed interpersonal relationships in the same way as other persons did. My personal experience with them even once convinced me that I am not a stigmatizer and I will never be one; it had almost made me agree that stigma is just a consequence of people's ignorance of patients, if not the ignorance of the diseases. I also turned to believe that close daily contact with patients may be an effective way to remove the stigma associated with these diseases. But, all of a sudden, Tianyu appeared to have challenged what I had imagined and believed, and even made me question who I am, what kind of person I am and what I will do in the face of people who are different. Tianyu has challenged what I believed stigma is actually about. I started wondering whether or not I would really care to know about these individuals or would have made contact with them, if I had not been doing this research. At that moment I guessed that my answer would be the same as many of my healthy friends, who would ask in reply, "Why would I want to do that?"

I began reflecting on my own feeling about and my responses to Tianyu. I asked myself why I would feel annoyed and harassed by Tianyu. Apparently, it was not because of his AIDS, otherwise I would have felt the same way with the other HIV/AIDS patients; it was not because of his mental illness either, which had never been diagnosed. Instead, it was because he acted as if he had no sense at all about how to engage appropriately in interpersonal relationships. He spoke of everything but had no sense about what he should or should not say under certain circumstance. He had no sense of shame, talking about sex in detail in front of me. He had no idea about the formal relationship between him and me, between a patient and a volunteer or researcher; he kept staring at me and following me; he touched me without the sense about what bodily contact means in Chinese culture; without knowing whether or not I am a gay, which he seemed not to care to know. He even wanted to jiaowang with me and considered me a potential lover who he could develop a relationship with. All he had done to me together with his AIDS identity combined to make me feel annoyed and harassed. If Tianyu was not an AIDS patient but acted this way in front of me, I would have the same feeling about him; however, his AIDS identity definitely made how I felt about him even worse. For me, he was absolutely bu dong shi: He was not aware of his own identity; he had no idea about his own position or status in the interpersonal relationship between him and me. He said to me what he should not have said; he acted in the way he was not supposed to. He had absolutely crossed the line. That was why I felt offended and annoyed. In fact, a person who is considered bu dong shi and does not know how to engage appropriately in relationships is often called shenjingbing (the mentally ill) in Chinese context, no matter whether or not the person really has a mental illness. Reversely, this fact also suggests how the mentally ill are perceived in Chinese context: they are considered non-persons, who are basically unable to engage appropriately in interpersonal relationships centered on social life, which means they are unable to build their own social networks and live effectively in the social world.

During that weekend, Tianyu kept sending me text messages through his cell phone. Some of his messages are quoted here:

On Sunday 12:48 pm, "Thank you for your concern about me. Hope we can become good friends."

13:05 pm, "Guo, this is our predestined affinity. I will be happy every day. Your friend, Tianyu."

22:45, "Guo, my brother scolded me again. I cannot take it anymore. I really want to go to your place. I am crying in my heart."

22:52 pm, "I really cannot take it anymore."

I did reply to each of these messages, but what I said back to him was nothing further than just trying to comfort him. I had to admit that I would have responded more actively if I did not feel offended and annoyed with him. In addition, given what I had heard from Mrs. Ding about Tianyu's being a liar, I came to suspect every word I heard from him. I believed that his brother scolded and abused him, but I simply doubted that he really needed immediate help at that moment. Instead, I took his words as both overreaction and a manipulating technique he had developed to attract attention. Hence I assumed that nothing necessary needed to be done. I instinctively responded that way to Tianyu's call for help. Later I realized how categorizing someone as a non-person could easily result in ignoring that person's suffering and damaging that person's credibility. The identity of non-person simply makes people's indifference to the non-person's suffering legitimate and reasonable. The reason I did not feel offended or annoyed with Zhanshan and other patients was that they did not say or do anything like Tianyu did to me. They were not non-persons in my eyes. But for their families, what they were and had done was apparently not the same as it meant to me. In the perspective of their families, they are non-persons.

The next Monday, I had a talk with Mrs. Ding and Zhanshan about Tianyu at the AIDS Care Center. Mrs. Ding told me that Tianyu called her the night before, saying he had a good talk with me. She felt happy that I liked to talk with Tianyu; also, she was glad to have someone else who could share the burden that Tianyu had put on her shoulders. She told me that Tianyu had been calling her from morning to late night almost every day, regarding all kinds of trivial things. She did not mean to complain about it, but I could tell that she was definitely exhausted and did not have a clue how to deal with this situation. Mrs. Ding said that Tianyu's brain was not clear; she thought that it might be caused by some provoking events that happened to him at home. She also mentioned that Tianyu's birth father and mother were close relatives and suggested that he might have inherited certain brain problems and his brother seemed to have similar problems. After Tianyu's father and mother divorced, his mother married again. She moved out to live with her new husband but left Tianyu and his brother behind. Occasionally she would visit Tianyu and his brother and give them a little money and food. In addition, Tianyu and his brother received 200 yuan each year distributed by the local street community.

"That is all they have. His brother does not have a job either. I don't know how they can make a living by that. They are really miserable. But Tianyu has a strong sense of self-esteem. He told me that his mother visited them frequently and often brought them money and food. As far as I know from his mother, that is not true. There was one time I heard from Tianyu that he was collecting cans in the streets to make money. He would not tell me about it, but that time he was too excited to control his own mouth," Mrs. Ding said.

Zhanshan stepped in, "His brother is a shenjingbing too. They are both shenjingbing." And then Zhanshan told me a story. Tianyu's brother once visited the Center and told everybody that he was busy all the time and had to work till late night every day. He felt sorry that he could not make any time for his brother, but he was happy that the Center could help him take care of his brother. He even promised Mrs. Ding that he would like to pay the Center 1000 yuan each month for taking care of his brother.

Out of the concern about where he could obtain that money, Zhanshan asked Tianyu's brother what he was doing, Tianyu's brother said he was working in a supermarket and there were only two staff working at night. He was working on the second floor and the other was on the first floor. Zhanshan burst into laughter, "Ha! He is just a security staff working a night shift in a supermarket." Zhanshan spoke of this event as a joke; he believed that Tianyu's brother was just boasting about his minor job. "The two brothers both like to boast," Zhanshan added, "They are both shenjing-bing. Ha!"

In order to show what kind of shenjingbing Tianyu is, Zhanshan told me another story of Tianyu's experience of finding a job. Tianyu was once hired by a company as a security staff member. In the beginning, he was required to attend a training session. On the second day of the training, he was late and missed most of the session. Hence he was asked to attend an extra session to make it up. But for no reason he became extremely angry and refused to do so, and then he was fired. "You tell me whether or not he is really a shenjingbing," Zhanshan laughed.

"What has troubled me most is that Tianyu is such a liar," Mrs. Ding said, "He often lies to attract your attention. We once organized an outing. Tianyuan also attended this activity. A patient made fun of him and said that he is too gay and does not look like a man. He was irritated and tried to climb a tree to show his masculinity. We could not stop him, and he fell down. Fortunately, the tree was not tall at all and he just had his arms scratched. But he insisted that his arm was broken. We had several doctors with us at that time; they immediately checked his arms and found there was nothing but scratches. But Tianyu wailed throughout that day. He didn't stop doing so even after that day. He called me several times, saying his arm was broken; he told everybody at the clinic that he had a broken arm," Mrs. Ding shook her head, "Mei banfa, I just feel that I cannot handle it anymore." Mrs. Ding preferred to use chaojia (squabble) and dajia (fight) to describe the conflicts between Tianyu and his brother, which Tianyu spoke of as discrimination and abuse. She said that Tianyu was not the only one who complained to her, and his brother also called her from time to time to complain about Tianyu. Mrs. Ding also told me that Tianyu once called her, saying his brother might have contracted AIDS too. "He sounded really happy when he said so to me. I just could not believe it, but

I was sure that he was lying again; he just wanted to say so as in act of revenge to disgrace his brother. The two brothers really give me a headache."

Tianyu showed up at the clinic around the lunch time that day. Mrs. Ding bought him lunch from the hospital's cafeteria. Given Tianyu's difficult financial situation, a free lunch could be really helpful for him. In contrast to the AIDS patients I met in Yunnan, most of the AIDS patients I met in Beijing were gay men and seemed to have been in much better financial situation. Many of them owned their own cars, which was not very common among average Chinese. But Tianyu was an exception. In addition to his well-known "brain problem," his poor financial situation also made him a definite "other" among the group. The way he dressed and ate both became jokes among the patient group. I heard many patients making fun of the way Tianyu ate. "He eats a lot. He eats as if he has not had food for years." During my stay at the Center, sometimes I invited several patients out for lunch or dinner. The last thing the other patients wanted to do was to take Tianyu with us to the meal; when Tianyu joined us, nobody wanted to sit beside him at the table; once he started eating, he would not stop for a second. In the end, he always complained that he was not full yet when everybody else already had enough. Hence I had to order one or two extra dishes only for him, and then everyone watched him eating till he finished it. In general, if a Chinese does so in a banquet, he/she will be considered bu dong li (not knowing courtesy), which directly causes not only the person but also the other persons at the same table to lose face (diu lian). It is not just an issue of bad banquet manners; instead, it is a comment on the sense of being a moral person. Given the fact that Tianyu's financial situation was so poor that he could not even afford meals by himself, I had no problem to forgive him at that time. Moreover, considering that my field work was just a short episode in my life and I would not have to witness and live with Tianyu's disturbing behavior day to day in the future, what kind of person he is would not be a long-term concern or worry for me. However, the other patients were apparently in a different situation and did not take it my way. Those patients had been together in the group for many years; they also knew about Tianyu's poor financial situation. They might not consider it a big deal at the very beginning. But after years watching Tianyu, his repetitive misbehavior became more and more unbearable for them. Sympathy came to be replaced completely by loathing; tolerance gradually progressed into hatred. Tianyu was stigmatized and discriminated against even within the AIDS group, among patients who had also contracted AIDS through homosexual intercourse.

With respect to stigma in the AIDS group, there is no doubt that the entire group has be divided into several subgroups in terms of different infections routes (blood transfusion, blood selling, heterosexual intercourse, homosexual intercourse, and sharing needles in using drug); moreover, based on different infection routes, these subgroups are morally categorized and constitute different levels of a hierarchical system. A widely accepted opinion among the general population is that the patients who contracted AIDS through blood transfusion are the most innocent victims for whom the health care system should be blamed; blood sellers are the second most innocent, for whom local governments and medical institutions should take the responsibility; at the bottom of the hierarchical categorization are the rest, who should blame themselves for their own wrong doing. However, this is just a view from the perspective of the society and may not be shared by the subgroups among the HIV/AIDS patients. As far as I observed, the view of innocence is only shared by the first three subgroups: Blood transfusion, blood selling and heterosexual intercourse groups. Gay men and drug users both believed that everyone who contracted AIDS is innocent and there is no difference on this issue between different subgroups: Gay men stated what society saw as wrongdoing they did for brave love; drug users believed that they shared the needles to HIV not out of reckless actions, but for the reason of unselfish friendship. In their opinions, blood sellers should be disdained for making money by selling blood; when it comes to the patients who contracted AIDS through blood transfusion, the members of other groups simply ignored the issue of innocence and asked in reply, "Who is not innocent? We are all innocent; we are all victims." Gay men and drug users both disdained each other and referred to the other as non-persons: Gay men described drug users as non-persons who were so addicted and selfish that they lost control of themselves and lost their own families; drug users teased gay men as bu nan bu nu (neither man nor woman) whose ambiguous gender identity constituted a source of shame for themselves and their families.

It is noteworthy that the word "innocence" is not completely refused use within the gay group among AIDS patients. They still speak of "innocence" when they refer to each other. Those who had a single partner, as they claimed, but still contracted AIDS often blamed their partner's unloyalty and considered themselves innocent; while the others tended to suspect those who claimed a single partner as a liar. Besides gay men, the patient group at the AIDS Care Center also had several members who contracted AIDS through other infection routes, such as heterosexual intercourse and blood transfusion. The gay group seemed to have a good relationship with these patients; some of them were close friends. For Tianyu, the other gay men did not consider him a real gay at all. Instead, they spoke of him as a retarded shenjingbing who was easily taken advantage of. Owing to Tianyu's suspicious gay identity, the other gay men within the patient group had never included him in their own group. Tianyu's problematic gay identity was not the only reason that he was stigmatized and excluded from this group, but it combined with his mentally ill behavior to make the entire patient group believe that he was nothing but mad.

There was an English language seminar at the Center, which was organized as a regular activity to help the patients keep in touch with each other and support each other. It turned out that Tianyu did not know about this seminar. When he found out that, he started complaining to Mrs. Ding and blaming her for not telling him. Mrs. Ding felt embarrassed and tried to explain to Tianyu. She said that she was so busy that she might have forgotten to inform him about the seminar. Tianyu was not satisfied with this explanation; he simply could not take the fact that he was forgotten and left behind. Later Mrs. Ding explained to me why she did not tell Tianyu about the seminar. Everyone who attended this seminar had to buy a textbook, which was more than 70 yuan; Mrs. Ding did not believe that that Tianyu could afford it, given his poor financial situation. "I know that sometimes he does not even have the money to take the bus. Where can he get the money for that book? He has a cell phone, but it is often inaccessible because of insufficient funds. Sometimes when he calls me, I really have a hard time to decide if I should answer it. If I do, I am afraid that it is just wasting his money; if I do not, I worry that something bad might have happened to him. But most of the time, he just talks about unnecessary things on the phone." In addition to her worry about Tianyu's financial situation; Mrs. Ding had another concern, "Tianyun really has some problem with his brain, and he often ruins these activities. He just does not fit in under such circumstance. Many patients do not like him. Some of them even told me that they would not attend the seminar if Tianyu was going to be there. He is not suitable to these things. The entire atmosphere would have changed if he joined us."

That day, Tianyu still followed me everywhere at the Center, following me after work to take the same bus till he had to transfer to another one. On the bus, he told me in a happy mood, "I reported my brother to my mother. My mother blamed my brother for scolding and beating me; she threatened to remove him from our family resident registry booklet (hukouben)." To remove someone from the family resident registry booklet means to officially remove the person from his family, indicating the person is not considered a family member anymore. Tianyu seemed to have been gloating at his brother's misfortune. He was really happy with his mother's reaction to his brother. But I was not sure if he was telling truth. Did he just make up his mother's words to make himself feel better? I did not know; I just felt that his story was unaccountable, his words were unreliable, and he was really annoying.

When I later recalled about Tianyu's being excluded from that English language seminar, I was surprised to find that I did not feel sympathy toward Tianyu. Although I could not agree with Mrs. Ding not to tell Tianyu about the seminar, neither did I consider her decision to exclude Tianyu from the seminar morally incorrect. I believed that my feeling at that moment had much to do with my own personal experience with Tianyu; it resulted from the poor interpersonal relationship between Tianyu and me. I found myself more and more identifying with Mrs. Ding and the other patients, I did not like Tianyu either; I felt annoyed by him and wanted to get away from him. Tianyu did not sense the fullness of my reaction to him. During the next several days, he showed up at the Center every day and kept me company, followed me everywhere; after work, he still took the same bus as I did; he still kept sending me text messages or calling me. I just felt that I did not have much to talk with him about; I tried to reply to each of the messages he sent to me but no longer took them seriously. After a week I could not take it anymore. At the Center, I started avoiding him and spending more time with the other patients; after work, I began ignoring some of his phone calls and text messages and delaying my replies. Eventually Tianyu came to realize the change. Although he still accompanied and followed me, he did not do it the way he did before. I did not feel sorry at all for what I had done to him; instead I felt relieved.

On Thursday of the next week, Tianyu did not show up at the Center until 5 pm. Upon walking into the Center, he began complaining. He went to a company for a job interview that morning. But the company wanted someone younger than 25. Since Tianyu was already older than 30, the company would not hire him. He complained to me, "They have problem with their own eyes. How could they tell that I am older than 30? Do I look like older than 30? They were just wasting my time."

"But you are older than 30, aren't you? I remember that you told me about it, didn't you?" I was a little confused.

"Yes. That is correct." Tianyu replied.

I was even more confused, "Then how did they get to know about your age?"

"They asked me about it, and then I told them." He said in anger.

Tianyu was not angry with the company's rule of not hiring people older than 25; instead, he was angry with the fact that the company found him to be older than 30. But the truth is that he was older than 30, moreover he told the company himself about his age. I did not understand where his anger was coming from; his complaint did not make any sense to me at all. But soon my confusion left me. I told myself, "He has a brain or mental problem. He did not even know what he was talking about. It is normal that his talk does not make any sense. The company might also find this out during the interview. Why would they hire such a person?" I stopped responding to his narrative and began ignoring his complaining. More and more, I came to have the same feeling as the other patients had about Tianyu: a retarded shenjingbing. Later, Mrs. Ding had Tianyu diagnosed by a psychiatrist; it turned out that Tianyu had both affective disorder and cognitive failure. None seemed to care much about this diagnosis because Tianyu was already considered and treated as a mentally ill even without the diagnosis. In one of his articles, Corrigan (2007) describes how clinical diagnosis might exacerbate the stigma of mental illness. In his view, diagnostic label and social stereotype combine to intensify prejudice, and then lead to discrimination against the mentally ill. Corrigan also believes that "contact between the public and people with mental illness leads to significant change in the stereotypes about mental illness" and "contact counters stigma by highlighting people as individuals with complex lives that exceed the narrow descriptions of diagnosis" (2007: 36). Hence, he proposes that "regular contact with people with mental illness and focusing on recovery may diminish the stigmatizing effects of diagnosis" (2007: 31). My personal experiences with Zhanshan and other HIV/AIDS patients have approved Corrigan's point: My daily contact with them revealed to me that each of them was not just an AIDS patient but a whole person with "complex life"; but my experience with Tianyu definitely approved the opposite: it was in my "regular contact" with him that I developed my stigmatizing attitude against him. Stigma is definitely related to the public stereotype of the stigmatized group. The question is what if the public do not care to know about this individual's entire lives other than the stereotype. In fact, for most people in a society, either the mentally ill or the HIV/AIDS patients are nothing but an imagined community; the general public simply have no regular contact with these individuals, let alone whether or not they want to know about them.

During that period, I often reflected on the way I treated Tianyu. I asked myself if I became one of those patients who stigmatized and discriminated against Tianyu, or if I was one of them from the very beginning and Tianyu's appearance exposed my true nature of being a stigmatizer. In either situation, I could not convince myself that I was not. As a researcher, I was supposed to take an objective stance and avoid over-involvement with my informants. However, for my anthropological involvement in the field, especially focusing on such a topic as stigma, I found that I could hardly have myself involved in a calm and objective way. I could hardly detach myself from my personal values, moral sense and emotions. After all, I was still one of the persons who was living in the same local context and instinctively applied the local moral sense to whoever I met. On the other hand, both my anthropological training and the ethical sense behind the goal of my research forced me to constantly rethink my involvement in the field, examine what I had done to research subjects, and remind myself that I should have acted as an objective outsider. However, by retaining my identity of researcher and keeping a certain distance from research subjects, I often found that I could easily become the object I opposed in an ethical sense. I have been through a struggle in my inner world since I started my field work. Tianyu was the one who made me rethink this struggle most powerfully. The struggle was not just the conflict between the double-identities of a researcher: Both a researcher and a local person; it was also the conflict between the professional obligation of a researcher and ethical sense from which a suffering witness cannot escape. Although this struggle had been bothering me from time to time, one thing I am sure about is that my personal experience, especially with Tianyu, was able to show me how a patient's AIDS and mental illness status combined with his failure in engaging appropriately in interpersonal relationships to result in his being stigmatized among the general public to which I belong, and even within AIDS patient group.

Comparison Located in Local Context

My ethnography on mental illness and HIV/AIDS shows that, in both cases, stigma is embodied in similar areas: subjects are stigmatized within institutions, including schools, work units and other government institutions; they are stigmatized within the health care system; they are stigmatized within the local communities, such as village and neighborhoods; they are stigmatized among relatives and within families. Stigmatization is also actualized in similar ways: the subjects are avoided, ignored, teased, blamed, accused, abandoned, and even killed in the most extreme case. The main reason I quoted Tianyu's case in this chapter is to make a comparison between the stigma associated with mental illness and that associated with HIV/AIDS. It is noteworthy that the comparison I am talking here about aims at the stigma in local context, rather than public stigma, which psychologists and experts in public health usually refer to.

Volinn (1989) compares leprosy stigma to AIDS stigma in terms of the two diseases' definitions and their implications. Volinn's comparison is based on the epidemiological and etiological characteristics of the two diseases, including "the impairment, disability and handicap, implications of these labels and the importance of additional categorization of the morbidity condition" (1989: 1157). Volinn argues that "the question of contagiousness and the relative risk is particularly important as far as social reactions are concerned" and "perception for risk contributes to the social construct of illness". For leprosy, "exact identification of risk is still indeterminate", but "that factor of ambiguity is a definite contributor to stigma assigned the disease" (1989: 1160). For AIDS, "roots of stigmatization can be traced to traditional commitment to values of monogamous family unit, and to the consideration of homosexuality as either immorality or a disease to be treated through practice of psychiatry or psychoanalysis" (1989: 1161). Volinn starts from the two diseases' epidemiological and etiological characteristics and ends up emphasizing social perception of the two diseases, but she applies two different approaches to compare the two situations: Risk analysis to leprosy and causal attribution to AIDS. That double standard makes the distinction between leprosy stigma and AIDS stigma more a product of her own research method. In addition, without ethnographic evidences, simply differentiating leprosy stigma from AIDS stigma in terms of imagined general social beliefs will not be able to help us understand the deep "implications" associated with the two illnesses.

Walkey *et al.* (1990) attribute stigma associated with AIDS to a new and negative stereotype, compared to stigma related to mental illness. They argue that stigma related to mental illness is caused by "common fears and anxiety induced by serious biological and psychological dysfunction" (1990: 552); while, in the case of AIDS, moral denigration adds to these common fears and anxiety, and then creates the stereotype of AIDS, which is the very reason that the AIDS patients are stigmatized against. They consider stigma a static social attitude; moreover, they seem to believe that "moral denigration" is involved in the case of AIDS but not in the case of mental illness.

Mak *et al.* (2006) conducted quantitative research on comparative stigma in Hong Kong. By using a telephone survey, they compared public stigma toward three diseases: SARS, TB and HIV/AIDS. "Findings showed that public stigma was the highest towards HIV/AIDS, followed by TB and SARS". Among the general population, many people who have no direct contact with these subjects have to either imagine these subjects or simply reply as are socially desired. This method may be effective to display public attitude on stigma across different diseases. However, without considering the local context, simply reducing stigma into a generalized public attitude that can be measured by questionnaires will not be able to reveal the stigma in reality.

As I already stated, I felt annoyed with Tianyu and began avoiding him not because of his AIDS status, but because of his failure, caused by mental illness, to engage appropriately in interpersonal relationships. Tianyu was stigmatized within the AIDS group because he was considered a retarded shenjingbing. The two facts seemed to suggest that the stigma associated with mental illness is even stronger than the one associated with HIV/AIDS in China, but jumping to that conclusion from the two facts can be problematic. It is easy to find the opposite example. Just imagine if Tianyu was in a group of the mentally ill, there will be no doubt that he would be stigmatized within that group too because of his gay identity and AIDS status. Neither example proves which stigma is stronger. Hence, the question is not just which, mental illness or HIV/AIDS, matters more; but also to whom it matters. The first fact, my response to Tianyu, further approves this point: to whom it matters. Tianyu's AIDS does not matter much to me, but it does matter to his family; while his failure in engaging appropriately in interpersonal relationships, compared to his AIDS status, apparently matters more to me due to the daily contact and interaction between Tianyu and me. As I already analyzed, Zhanshan and the other patients' AIDS status might not be a concern or bother for me, but it meant a lot to their own families.

To whom it matters implies that it will be difficult to compare the stigma related to mental illness with that related to HIV/AIDS without considering whom the audiences are and how they are involved. It also suggests that the difference of degree might not be a valid perspective to explore the difference of stigma between the two situations. Extra explanation is needed here to further make this point. The question goes this way: As far as the same audience is concerned, is it possible to compare the two situations in terms of difference in the degree of stigma? Firstly, based on the real life world, anthropological field work is different from the natural sciences because it is impossible to do experiments: such as place a mentally ill person in a family and observe how the family responds to him or her, and then put an HIV/AIDS patient into the same family, apply the same observation, and then make a comparative study. In reality, although I happened to have met a patient who had both mental illness and AIDS, it is difficult to find such cases in the field. Even if I could find a sample of such case, there would be no way to observe how the family reacted to the two situations independently, the mutual influence and inter-correlation between the two situations cannot be ignored. Therefore, what I can do is to compare how the mentally ill and the HIV/AIDS patients were responded to within their respective families.

Feldman *et al.* (1999) conducted research to explore whether the medical professionals in the United States and China adhere to different ethical standards. They found "significant differences in clinical ethical beliefs between internists in the United States and China, most evident in informing patients of a cancer diagnosis. In general, the Chinese physicians appeared to give far greater weight family preference in medical decision than did the U.S. physicians" even "when family members' wishes conflicted with a patient's preferences" (1999: 469). Their research aimed at the ethical standards within health care system across different cultures, but it showed how family was involved in patients' illness experience in China. It also suggested that, in Chinese context, a person is first and foremost a family member rather than an independent individual. Stigma related to mental illness and HIV/AIDS makes it even clear that a disease is not just about a psychical or psychological problem to an individual but illness experiences of the patient and his/her family. Given that, for a research focusing on stigma as I conducted in China, a stigmatized person has to be taken into account at first in the context of family.

A look back at the cases I include in chapters two, three and four indicates that stigmatization within the family is only mentioned in one case of the mentally ill; while stigmatization of the HIV/AIDS patients within their families are almost present in every case. A mentally ill person I included in chapter two was blamed for feigning illness; while the HIV/AIDS patients appearing in chapters three and four were scolded, accused, even abandoned and left to die by their families. These facts might give readers an impression: the HIV/AIDS patients were more stigmatized than the mentally ill within their families; or stigma related to HIV/AIDS is much stronger than that associated with mental illness. This impression, I have to clarify, has much to do with both the limited sample included in the mental illness part and the major site, hospitals, where I choose to conduct my research. During my field work on mental illness, all of the patients I interviewed were suffering relatively minor mental illnesses, such as depression and anxiety disorder. I was not allowed to meet or interview patients with most severe mental illnesses, who were considered dangerous and all locked up in isolated buildings; moreover, they were assumed by medical professionals to be unable to communicate with others. In addition, for research aimed at mentally ill and HIV/AIDS patients, I was not allowed to conduct my research as most of anthropologists have done in their research: staying in a local community, such as a village or an urban neighborhood, and conducting long-term participant observation. Considering my research subjects, I was not allowed to go to a local community and look around for these patients, which would violate the protection of human subject requirement. Hence hospital became the major site where I could gain access to research subjects. This limitation resulted in my inability to present the entire range of stigma related to mental illness in this research. However, the fact that the patients with most severe mental illnesses were isolated and inaccessible still displays how strong stigma related to mental illness is. In addition to the fact that the mentally ill persons I met at the hospital were suffering relatively minor mental illnesses, most of them were young and in the early phase of the course of their illnesses, when their families had not given up on them but still cared enough to try to seek treatment for them in hope that they could recover soon and completely. Even so, I still witnessed how their families complained about them and blamed them for not recovering, for repetitive relapse and even for feigning illness.

In fact, cases in which the mentally ill are left uncared for and even abandoned by their families are not rare in China. According to data from Chinese Health Ministry, the mentally ill in China are estimated at around 16 million. By the end of 2006, China had 19,130 psychiatrists in total, of which less than 20% had received professional training, and 145,570 ward beds for the mentally ill. Of the mentally ill less than 10% are receiving treatment (Zhang 2006). Given the huge gap between need and supply, it is not difficult to imagine how many mentally ill persons are left without care. In Tianjing, among 360 mentally ill who had been hospitalized at a local hospital longer than a year, 99 received little care from their families, and 49 were abandoned by their families (Zhou and Cao 2004). Kohrman (1999), in his study of que zi (the lame), analyzes how marriage exclusion caused by disability compromises the identity formation among disabled men in China. He cited the case of the physically disabled Ah Bo, who went through several arranged dating meetings set up by his brother and sister-in-law. None of these meeting worked out for him. In the end, his brother and sister-in-law became "more and more irritated at Ah Bo for not fulfilling the expectation of having a spouse contributing to the joint family's housework" (2000: 896). After "a series of squabbles", Ah Bo and his mother was forced to "move out of the family's sprawling, white-stucco house and into a dark, small, brick hut" (2000: 897). He was abandoned by his brother and sister-in-law. Ah Bo's story shows that even a physically disabled man could be so stigmatized within the family that he was kicked out. Hence, even the stigma related to disability within family can also progress to its ultimate phase: abandonment.

In a sense, stigma across different illnesses in the local context can hardly be measured or compared to each other in terms of degree. Kohrman's research suggests that, no matter to what diseases it is related, stigma is likely to progress along with the worsening of the interpersonal relationships within the family toward its extreme phase: the family abandons the stigmatized. Therefore, stigma related to mental illness and that related to HIV/AIDS can both progress to the extreme phase within the family: abandoning and otherwise getting rid of the stigmatized, psychically and physically.

Alonzo and Reynolds (1995) argue that stigma has to be considered as "changing and emerging over the course of a single disease". They analyze stigma related to HIV/AIDS in terms of the disease trajectory and describe how stigma is "affected by changes in the biophysical dimensions of HIV/AIDS". They point out four phases of the HIV/AIDS stigma trajectory: "(1) at risk: pre-stigma and the worried well; (2) diagnosis: confronting an altered identity; (3) latent: living between illness and health; and (4) manifest: passage to social and physical death" (1995: 303). Alonzo and Reynolds replace stigma into a dynamic framework; however, their stigma trajectory theory is based on pathological trajectory of disease and from an individual perspective of HIV/AIDS patients. As I observed in field work, the dynamics of stigma have to be taken into account in the context of family, community and society.

Kohrman's research and many cases I found in field work showed that, in the real life world, stigma is dynamic: always changing and progressing alongside the involvement of patients, their families, local communities and broader society in dealing with the critical situation brought about by illness. In Ah Bo's story, his brother and sister-in-law started by helping him find a wife but ended up accusing and abandoning him. In my field work, most families with mentally ill members have experienced several phases of stigma over the course of the illness. As the illness developed, the entire family often engaged the painful journey: seeking treatment for the patient, witnessing repetitive relapse, complaining and accusing the patient, feeling hopeless, putting the patient in a mental hospital, and abandoning the patient in the end. Therefore, stigma has to be considered in a social dynamic framework. This point of view directly leads to the question: what does mobilize this dynamic process?

Moral Common Sense Behind Stigma in China — What Makes a Human or Person

Stigma implies a strong emotion rather than an attitude resulting from risk perception and calculation; this emotion comes from its local moral meaning and daily practices. Yang *et al.* (2007) point out that stigma is "an essentially moral issue" and "a moral experience" concerning about "what really matters and what is threatened" in a local world (2007: 1524). In this sense, stigma is the embodiment of the local moral meaning; it is created, maintained and supported by the local moral world and the meaning it assigns to certain human conditions. On the other hand, this emotion and the local moral meaning behind it have been fostered and strengthened by stigmatization. Stigma is a consequence of applying local moral common sense and sensibility to these subjects, rather than a misconduct of moral denigration. Hence, it is considered legitimate, reasonable and, more importantly, morally correct in the local context. Both mentally ill and the HIV/AIDS patients are considered non-persons in terms of local moral meaning, which is the very reason why they are treated as non-persons, deprived of their basic human rights, and excluded from formal institutions, local communities, and even their families. Hence, to explore the difference between the two, one has to analyze the moral meanings about personhood behind these two serious health conditions.

In the Chinese view, no one is born a human or a person. That is to say, no one is born with the right to be a human or person; instead, one has to learn to be a human first in the context of the family and then a person in society, and also to act as a person to prove his/her personhood. Being a person can only be achieved through zuo ren (acting as a person), which means one has to show others that he/she is a person by acting as a person: showing and proving one's ability to be a person by engaging appropriately in interpersonal relationships, establishing social relationships and building social networks. Acting like a person makes a person.

Chinese people refer both human and person to ren. Yet there is a clear distinction when they refer to ren between those who are only accepted by their families and those who are accepted by the society, including their families. Here I call the former human and the latter person for sense of differentiation. Accordingly, I call a person without social acceptance a non-person while a person without family acceptance a non-human. A person who cares for nothing but his/her own family, or a person who cares for his/her family but is unable to engage in interpersonal relationships or to build social networks outside of the family is actually not a person but a non-person in the eyes of society, but he/she is still seen as a person within family. When a person is rejected and abandoned by his/her family, either the family is blamed for inhumanness if the person is not at fault, or the person is accused of being a non-human for what he/she did to the family. But there is the third situation in which no one is to blame, which can be observed in the most extreme cases of taking care of family members with psychosis. In such cases, families often spend years even decades taking care of their sick members; in the end they have to give up on the patient. Kleinman and Lin (1981) described how love has changed to denial and rejection in this process. In this situation, no one is to blame, but that does not change the fact that the member who is rejected and abandoned by his/her family became a non-human who lost the last rights of being a human and the last protection, which is supposed to be provided by the family. Being a non-human in Chinese society means belonging nowhere and without rights, relationships or protections, which makes even the most aggressive or inhuman treatment to the person blameless. Non-human condition makes the extreme stigmatizing situation possible and legitimate.

1. From non-person to non-human

In the case of mental illness, there is a significant distinction between the rural (or traditional) view and the urban (or modern) view on the genesis of mental illness. The former considers mental illness a dirty disease: Patients are either polluted or possessed by dirty things (ghosts in general), which is a punishment for what they did in the past; the latter tends to attribute mental illness to the personal stress created by increasing and overwhelming social pressure and one's failure in adjusting to the changing society. However, both views have one point in common, which is that mental illness is not biologically or genetically determined; instead, a person can only be driven crazy either by his/her family members or by tragic family events. Hence, mental illness implies the existence of family grievance, meaning something really wrong, generally concerning injustice within the family, is going on in the family. Family grievance means shame for the entire family. The shame binds the patient with his/her families so closely that the family instinctively tries to hide that they have a member with mental illness in order to save face for the entire family. Otherwise the grievance within the family will be exposed and the entire family has to face devastatingly negative moral judgment and social isolation in the local community.

To hide the shame, the family generally sends patient to hospitals that are far away to seek medical help secretly. They hide the situation from the local community, including their relatives, friends, neighbors and workmates. This process can be very painful; the family has to make up excuses to conceal what is really going on; they have to seek help secretly in another city, even another province; they are afraid to tell anyone, even the closest relatives or friends. They will not stop having the mentally ill person diagnosed again and again until they finally give up and accept the reality. After the diagnosis is confirmed, they start to search the best available hospitals for hospitalization. They have to deal with repetitive relapse. During the period of remission, they have to take care of the patient at home. In the end, the case of mental illness becomes impossibly to hide; it comes to be visible in the local community. As some people get to know about this family secret, the family still manages to hide it from other people. But the suspicion about the mentally ill member is eventually confirmed. His or her new identity, that of a mentally ill person, has become public and, in a sense, official. Having mental illness implies being a non-person, who is not assumed to be able to act as a normal person in the eyes of society. The entire family feels ashamed and begins retreating from the public sphere. For the mentally ill person, he or she probably has to quit school or work. If the patient is still young, his or her school or professional career is suspended immediately; it is very likely that the person will not find anyone to marry. There is no chance that the person can get back on the track of a normal life. The patient has to accept the fact that he or she will be considered and treated as a non-person from that moment on and that he or she is going to be separated and excluded from the local community for the rest of life.[1]

The patient soon loses all his/her social relationships because the local community simply considers him/her a non-person who already has (it is assumed) lost the ability to engage appropriately in interpersonal relationships and no longer has the ability to establish new interpersonal relationships or maintain social networks. The entire family has to endure the rumors and social isolation. Out of shame, the family has to keep the patient at home. If the patient has a psychotic mental illness, the family becomes a silent part of the local community. Within the family, members start complaining about each other, the patient is going to be blamed and accused, so he/she is stigmatized within the family itself. If the patient experiences violence as part of his/her mental illness, his/her dangerous behavior is soon going to be known within the local community. The patient is considered a danger to the local community, while the entire

[1] I am talking here about psychosis, not minor psychological problems.

family will be blamed and accused for any threat posed by the patient upon the local community. As the violent psychosis develops, the patient appears to no longer recognize other family members as such and starts attacking them. The family has no choice but to lock up the patient at home. As the patient becomes more and more dangerous to his/her own family, the family feels desperate and hopeless. The patient becomes a non-human in the eyes of the other family members for not recognizing family members and for attacking them. The family now has a good reason to abandon the patient in the name of protecting the rest of the family. Finally the patient is separated and excluded from his/her own family; so he/she loses the last interpersonal relationship, the connection to the family. The patient, who has been abandoned by his/her own family, becomes a non-human. A person without family is not just a non-person but non-human. That means, he/she has no rights, no agency, no protection at all. This is an extreme case. In fact, most mentally ill persons are not violent. Yet the cultural scenario of the fear of violence drives the societal experience toward the central concern of protecting the community, and away from primary concern with caring for the patient.

The mentally ill have been gradually driven out of all their social networks (first the local community and then the family) along with the progression of the illness. During that process, the patient's identity transforms from person to non-person, and then into non-human; at the same time, the stigma progresses to its extreme phase.

2. From non-human to non-person

Among the general population in China, HIV/AIDS was basically considered a foreign disease, which was transferred from foreign countries to China, and also a dirty disease caused by sexual deviance and drug abuse. Although many patients contracted HIV/AIDS through blood transfusion and blood selling in China, the Chinese people still link HIV/AIDS to sexual deviance or drug abuse. They do so almost instantly and with an instinctive response and reactively imagination. It is hard to deny that the stigma associated with HIV/AIDS in China has much to do with that related to sexual deviance and drug abuse. "The dominant discourses of HIV/AIDS in china are still morally-centered, and people living with HIV/AIDS are constructed as morally problematic others" (Zhou 2007: 293).

In the Chinese context, both sexual deviance and drug abuse are not just considered an issue related to personal life style or individual moral sense; instead, they both imply treachery to the family, which also applies to HIV/AIDS. That is to say, HIV/AIDS implies irrefutable evidence of treachery to the family. In the Chinese view, contracting HIV/AIDS itself suggests that a person already has betrayed his/her family and consequently leads to the patient no longer being considered a family member. Although HIV/AIDS is not as visible as mental illness to the public and is relatively easier to disguise from the local community, it is difficult to conceal it from other members within the family, especially the patient's spouse. Since HIV/AIDS implies treachery to the family, the first danger the HIV/AIDS patient has to face is that he/she might be abandoned by the family. That is to say, HIV/AIDS patients are very likely first to become non-human in their families.

In the case of mental illness, although the shame is shared by the entire family, the rest of the family members often feel more ashamed because they are believed to have driven a member crazy. The shame of HIV/AIDS is basically considered the patient's shame, but the patient brings this shame to the entire family and loses face for the entire family. Therefore, the family members might be the first who give up on the HIV/AIDS patient and exclude him/her from the family. Many patients divorced when their spouses came to know about their HIV/AIDS status. Some of them chose to live separately under the same roof. Out of shame, both the patients and their spouses try to hide the illness; they do not divorce for fear that the HIV/AIDS status will be exposed in the public. The marriage is already dead, but they pretend to live together in order to conceal the broken marriage and also HIV/AIDS from their parents, from other family members and from people outside the family.

Given the hatred toward the HIV/AIDS patients and the extremely stressful situation caused by double identity within the family, the broken marriage is not able to last long. If the patient is not kicked out of the family, he/she has to continue to play a role with a double identity, a non-human within the family while a normal person in the public. The patient has to endure being stigmatized within the family while in fact there may be no public stigma because HIV status is so easy to hide and not disclose. The patient lives as a non-human in front of close family members who know about their AIDS status, but acts as a person in front of the rest of family and also in the neighborhood and community.

Once family members cannot take this painful situation anymore, the patient very likely is going to be quickly excluded from the family. If HIV/AIDS patients are excluded from their families, it is going to be very difficult for them to pretend to be a normal person and maintain a normal life in the public without support from their families. They already have lost their rights to be a human living within their families, but they have to pretend to act as a normal person in public, which often becomes very stressful and an almost impossible mission. If their HIV/AIDS status is disclosed, it is certain that they will lose their jobs. Most of the HIV/AIDS patients cannot handle this stress or do not want to take the risk; hence, they chose to quit their jobs. The burden brought about by the illness and the stigma forces them to keep to themselves and not to make any close relationships within the work unit, the community or even with a former friend, because a close relationship implies high risk for disclosing their HIV/AIDS status. Therefore, they have to retreat from the public sphere and live alone. Gradually, they exclude themselves from all social networks and cut off all interpersonal relationships, so that they make themselves into non-persons in the community.

It is worth noting that people who contracted HIV/AIDS through using drugs are generally considered criminals who have committed a serious crime against their own family. They are also highly stigmatized in their own families. Drug users are often considered non-humans in the family once they are caught using drugs. Moreover, using drugs is not easy to hide from the public, especially for long-time drug users. Once their drug users' identity has been found out in the public, they soon become non-persons in society. For patients who contracted HIV/AIDS through blood transfusion or blood selling, most of them consider themselves innocent victims and tend to speak up about their AIDS status in the public in order to seek help. But even being innocent in their own minds and those of the public does not change the fact that they are regarded as non-persons. They are no longer considered to be able to be a person; their situation is similar to what happens to the mentally ill persons.

The mentally ill persons generally experience the process of moving from losing social relationships to losing family relationships, and their identities change from being a person to being a non-person and then finally onto being a non-human. In contrast, HIV/AIDS patients generally experience the reverse process, moving from losing family relationships to losing social relationships, their identities transition from being a person to being a non-human and then onto being a non-person.

Identity transformation displayed in the two processes is determined by the moral common sense of what makes a person or a human in Chinese society. To understand stigma associated with mental illness and that related to HIV/AIDS in China, one has to take seriously the cultural framing of what makes a human or person in Chinese society. This cultural framing suggests that stigma is not just a result of popular ignorance of diseases, but is more about local moral common sense concerning what really matters for being a human or person and what is threatened in family, community, and broader society by such human health conditions.

The two opposite trajectories demonstrate two different micro processes of stigmatization related respectively to mental illness and HIV/AIDS in the context of family and local community. In the case of mental illness, public stigma plays a major part and starts the process; in the case of HIV/AIDS, stigmatization within family has a profound and determinant influence on the patient's identity transformation, given the fact that most HIV/AIDS patients are invisible in society. The implication of this difference suggests that anti-stigma programs must recognize and aim at different targets in dealing with individual cases of these two distinctive conditions.

Focusing on the micro process of stigmatization in the context of family and local community is helpful to explore the moral common sense inherent in stigma, which is what makes a human or person in the Chinese view. The implication of being a non-human or a non-person for the subjects themselves is social exclusion; but, what is the implication for local communities and even the state with its governmental institutions? To answer that, one has to take the broader society into account, which means that the involvement of the state and governmental institutions in the process of stigmatization has to been understood.

Absence and Passivity: The Role of State and Governmental Institutions in Taking Care of Mentally Ill Persons

Many families' painful journey of fighting mental illness ends up as family tragedies. Families often find blame hard to accept; anyone who witnesses this journey would hardly blame these families. But, in the Chinese context, these tragedies have seldom been connected to the absence of the state and governmental institutions in mediating the process. Why do these journeys often end up as nothing other than tragedies within the family? Few commentators attribute it to the developing but still limited mental health care service in China and the stigma related to mental illness on account of which families of the mentally ill are unwilling to be associated with mental health care services. In fact, the limited mental health care service is also a result of stigma associated with mental illness. Behind the fact that mental health care is undeveloped in contrast to other health care services in China is the popular belief that taking care of mentally ill persons is first and foremost a family responsibility. Pearson (1995) pointed out that, in China, mental health care has always been considered a family responsibility, which had been officially stated in the law since the Qing Dynasty. The role of the state and governmental institutions is to supervise and urge families to implement this responsibility and punish them when they are considered not fulfilling their duties.

The public media in China sensationally and constantly broadcasts reports of violent behavior and even killings committed by the mentally ill and reports of "wu fengzi" (violent mentally ill persons) being killed by their families. I did not find such cases myself during my field work, because in fact such violence is not a routine part of psychosis, but I would like to quote two cases I found in public media to show how stigma related to mental illness can cause a serious consequence in the family without the intervention of the state and governmental institutions to counteract public misperception and media distortion of what mental illness really is like.

A murder was reported from a village in Yunnan Province in 2007. A father, with the help of his brother and oldest son, killed another son who had been suffering from schizophrenia since 2006. As the report showed, the victim had given his family a real headache. He ran around all the time; did not sleep at night; stole livestock from both his own family and neighbors, and then sold them for money; beat up his father; put poison into a neighbor's food. The family had been in a poor financial situation even before the son was diagnosed with schizophrenia. They could not afford the treatment or hospitalization at all. The entire family was under great pressure created by neighbors' blame and criticism. Out of the great shame and unbearable suffering, the father killed his mentally ill son with the help of his brother and oldest son. They used an iron chain to bind the victim, and then strangled him in turn to death. In the end, the three murderers were sentenced respectively to 10 years in prison. Neither the state nor any governmental institution showed up during the process in which the family needed help, but appeared as the judge and punisher only after the family had to use murder to end the suffering.

The second case is about an older sister's murder of her younger sister who had chronic psychosis. The family had three daughters. It had been a happy family until the second daughter, Juanjuan, had a high fever in 2001 when she was in the sixth year of elementary school. After Juanjuan recovered from the high fever, she became another person and started losing control of her temper from time to time. Sometimes she even beat the other family members and smashed furniture. In 2004, Juanjuan was diagnosed with psychosis. The family tried everything, including medication and surgery, nothing ever worked. The situation was getting even worse; Juanjuan became more and more violent. She broke everything at home; none of the furniture at home remained intact. The most horrible thing for her family was that they could not tell when she was going to break out in madness. There was no sign at all. She acted as a normal person until the minute she turned into another person, crazy and violent. She poked her father's eyes with a chopstick, which almost caused his blindness; she slashed her older sister, Tingting, with a kitchen knife and left a huge scar on the latter's head; she pushed her mother, Suzhen, to the ground and battered her forehead. In the process of helping Juanjuan have a bath, Tingting was bitten, beaten and kicked so terribly that her body was covered with scars. Juanjuan even stabbed neighbors and relatives with scissors. In public, Juanjuan often broke out all of a sudden into wildly uncontrollable acts. She once pushed an 80-year-old woman into a ditch. Owing to her violent behavior, the family often received phone calls from the police, who emphasized that it was the family's responsibility to control the patient and that they would bear the consequence of her violence.

Out of desperation, Yong, her father, locked up Juanjuan with an iron chain at home. In order to take care of Juanjuan, Tingting dropped out her school and stayed at home. She told one of her former classmates that she had been under great pressure and wanted to kill herself. In 2005, Tingting swallowed a whole bottle of sleeping pills and tried to kill herself. Fortunately she was found by her father in time and sent to the hospital. After three days in coma she was saved. Later she wrote in her online blog, "While we locked you (Juanjuan) up, we were locked up too. Every time you break out, I just feel that I am fed up with my life. I really hope that I can somehow free myself from all of these things." Gradually, Tingting became silent and unsocial. She wrote in her blog, "I do not know what happened to me. I do not want to cry in front of my family. But now I'm alone so I can cry. You (the parents) put all of your hearts into Juanjuan. But what about me? I spend all my time to take care of her. Who cares about me? Who cares about how I feel? I feel that I am abandoned. I feel so lonely." Tingting was later diagnosed with depression. Yong tried to seek help for Juanjuan from local government institutions, but none showed concern or offered help. What he received was just a 200 yuan subsidy from the local welfare bureau.

For six years, the family had spent all they had saved, 100,000 yuan, seeking help for Juanjuan. In addition, they sold their apartment and borrowed money from many relatives and friends. They had tried everything they could find or think of, albeit without success. In early 2007, Yong decided to divorce his wife so that his wife and the other two daughters could leave this hell and live a normal life. He wanted to sacrifice himself and put the entire burden on his own shoulders. His wife and the other two daughters refused to leave. They held each other and cried. Yong had no choice but to find a mental hospital to send Juanjuan to. He contacted four mental hospitals, the first three all refused to take Juanjuan in: the first one simply refused them once they found out Juanjuan's maniacal condition; the second would take Juanjuan in only if the family paid

3,000–5,000 yuan each month and sent someone over to take care of Juanjuan all the time; the third refused Juanjuan too, for fear of her violent behavior. The fourth hospital accepted Juanjuan and asked for 2,000 yuan each month. The amount of money required was enormous, but the family had no option.

In August, 2007, Yong received a phone call from the mental hospital. He was asked to come and take care of Juanjuan, because Juanjuan could not live by herself at all. When the family arrived at the hospital, they found that Juanjuan was in a terrible situation. "She looked so miserable!" Yong recalled later. Juanjuan was wearing nothing but a coat; there was a bloody scar on her wrists left by hand cuffs. She cried to her mother, "It hurts." The hospital staff told Yong that Juanjuan refused to eat anything in the last 10 days. Tingting offered to stay and take care of Juanjuan. Yong refused at first, "Look at her! If you stay here, you are going to be abnormal too." Tingting shouted out to Yong, "Then what are we going to do? You have to work; mama has to take care of the housework. Who else is going to take care of Juanjuan?" Yong had nothing to say, and then he reluctantly agreed. After Yong and his wife left the hospital, Tingting helped Juanjuan have a bath and changed her clothes. Late that night, Tingting called her father and said, "Juanjuan is so miserable. I found feces all over her body when I was showering her."

The next morning, Yong received a phone call from the police; he was informed that Tingting had killed Juanjuan and then reported herself to the police. Tingting used a pillow to suffocate Juanjuan. In the interrogation, Tingting said that she wanted to help Juanjuan escape from her suffering. "Now she does not have to suffer anymore," she said, "My family had been suffering a lot since Juanjuan had this disease. Every one of us, including Juanjuan herself, all felt tired. I am so tired after taking care of her for six years. I thought to kill her in order to help everyone in my family escape from this pain. I had this idea since 2006." That night, after killing her younger sister, Tingting called a friend, saying, "It has been six years. My family is relieved now. Finally, I did something for my family. I don't care about what is going to happen to me. I am glad that I have this chance to help my family."

Yong forgave Tingting for killing Juanjuan; he believed that Tingting did it out of a good intention (shan yi) rather than evil intention (e yi), which was to help Juanjuan and the rest of the family. "It was Juanjuan's terrible situation in the mental hospital that made Tingting decide to kill her in order to end her suffering," Yong Said. After Tingting was arrested by the police, more than 200 neighbors signed a joint letter and sent it to the local justice department, testifying that Tingting had always been a good person and asking for a minor penalty for her. In the end, Tingting was sentenced to just probation; she did not have to go to prison. The judge believed that the murder had to do with her depression caused by taking care of Juanjuan for years. Also he recognized that the family had to bear the great stigma of their daughter's condition.

Considering this case, as Juanjuan's maniacal condition developed, the family had lived through several phases: Seeking medical help, locking up Juanjuan at home, putting her in a mental hospital, and killing her in the end. This tragedy shows how much a family had suffered from taking care of a violent and uncontrollable mentally ill member. More importantly, it suggests how pain, exhaustion and stigma associated with mental illness had forced a girl to kill her mentally ill younger sister. The murder can hardly be attributed to the stigmatization of a mentally ill member within the family. On the contrary, this case matches the model of "the loving care" by which Kleinman and Lin (1981) refer to the "unfailing care" and even "lifelong devotion" that Chinese families often give to their sick members. In this case, killing was the embodiment of family love rather than hatred: Watching Juanjuan suffer made Tingting suffer too; Tingting could not let her younger sister continue to suffer and be treated inhumanely that way in the mental hospital. Out of desperation, she had no choice but to end her sister's life, which was the only way she could find to end her younger sister's suffering. And, of course, this case makes us ask where the governmental agencies of the state were until the court intervened at the bitter end.

What is also noteworthy in this case is the public responses. This case has caused fierce controversy since it was published. Two opposite points of view were expressed. Some people blamed Tingting for killing her younger sister and insisted that a murder was a murder and Tingting should have been put on trial for the murder; others had great sympathy for the entire family and pointed out that those who blamed Tingting had never experienced such unbearable suffering and did not have any idea about it. However, most people defined the event as nothing more than a family tragedy; a few of them blamed the mental health hospital for causing this murder or sighed about the backwardness of mental health care service in China; none ever questioned what else other than the disease had caused the desperate situation in the family or whether the state and governmental institutions should have done something about it before it turned to be a murder within the family. The way the public responded to this case suggests that, even in today's China, taking care of mentally ill persons is still considered a family duty, and through there is criticism of the passivity and ineffectiveness of institutions, they do not bear the chief blame, because the expectation is so low based on the reality, an absence of presence of helping institutions.

The tendency in traditional Chinese medicine to somatize mental disorders and consider them psychical diseases or symptoms of psychical disorders has a profound influence on both the public and medical professionals' view of mental illnesses in China (Lin 1985; Kleinman 1988). This view undermines the need of a special care system dealing with mental illness in the framework of traditional Chinese medicine. Moreover, in regard to mental illnesses, the concern about the possible disturbance and threat caused by mentally ill persons to the social order has been taking priority over the medical treatment of mental illness. In the Chinese history, locking up mentally ill persons had always been based on the concern about social security and stability rather than the treatment of mental illness in the medical sense (Yang *et al.* 2006: 76). In 1689, Daqing *luli* published by the Qing Dynasty stated that the families which have mentally ill members should report the patients to the local government and, at the same time, take the responsibility to lock up the patients at home. The local officials were demanded to distribute chains and fetters to these families for locking up the mentally ill members. If the families did not take their responsibility and thus the patients hurt or killed others, the families would be blamed and punished (Yang *et al.* 2006: 77). If the families unlocked the patients without notifying the local government, they would be punished too. Only if family or relatives were not available to take their responsibility, the local government would take it over and lock up the patients at official facilities (Yang *et al.* 2006: 77).

In the late 19th century, Western missionaries introduced mental health care to China. In 1872, one of the American missionaries, John Kerr, started to advocate the idea of "the ration treatment" in the hospitals managed by missionaries in China. In his efforts, the first mental hospital in China was established in Guangzhou city of Guangdong province in 1892. However, the hospital did not seem to work well: the death rate among the mentally ill persons who were hospitalized at the hospital was high and few patients really recovered from the ration treatment. The reason was that most of the patients who were sent to the hospital by their families were already at the last phase of their psychoses (Yang *et al.* 2006: 81). In this sense, the practice of this hospital and its idea of the ration treatment did not successfully change the Chinese view of mental illness and the way the Chinese families respond to their mentally ill members. Families still hid and locked up the mentally ill members at home for many years while seeking help privately. In the end when the patients became a threat to the local community and also a threat to the family's social status in the local community, the families felt exhausted and eventually gave up on the patients, and then they sent the patients to the hospital.

After 1949 when Chinese Communist Party took over the country, the health of the individual became symbolically intertwined with the health of the new regime (Heller 1973; Chang *et al.* 2002: 30). In contrast to the fact that sexually transmitted diseases, snail fever, bubonic plague, small pox, leprosy and cholera disappeared in a few years under the strong medical intervention from the state, mental health care had almost been suspended after 1949. On one hand, mental illnesses were politicized and considered the leftover of jiu shehui (old society), which was assumed only produced by evil social institutions, such as feudalism and capitalism, along with drug abuse and prostitution; while in the xin shehui (new society) established by its Chinese communist party there would be no more mental illnesses, even those mentally ill persons left by the old regime should automatically recover because of the establishment of new regime. This politicized view of mental illness directly led to the denial of the existence of mental illness and exclusion of mental illnesses from the concern of public health. On the other hand, "revolutionary zeal alone could not overcome the severe shortages in trained staff, inadequate facilities in most areas, limited economic resources" (Chang *et al.* 2002: 31).

During the Cultural Revolution, mental illnesses were connected with wrong political thinking (Pearson 1995) and were treated as political errors to be eliminated (Chang *et al.* 2002: 31); the label of mental illnesses was used as a weapon to delegitimize and attack political dissidents. After the Cultural Revolution, mental health care started to develop but at a slow pace and only in large cities in China.

In addition to the somatization of mental illnesses in traditional Chinese medicine theories, political and economic factors also shape the social perception of mental illness and the demand for mental health services (Chang *et al.* 2002: 31). "The focus of care is on preventing chronic patients from causing social disruption. Thus social control is valued in the care system, and there has been inadequate attention to patients' rights and their protection" (Chang *et al.* 2002: 31). In China, mental illnesses were not officially acknowledged to be among the most important public health problems until 1999 (Yin 2000). "For the first time statements were made to the effect that patients' rights must be respected" (Chang *et al.* 2002: 31). In current China, mental health care is mainly and increasingly focusing on psychological problems, while health care for people with psychosis is, with the exception of Beijing, Shanghai and several other large cities, left far behind. Three factors have contributed to this situation: first, the vast territory with enormous geographic, demographic, economic and cultural diversity results in the regionalization of mental health care; second, a shortage of trained mental health professionals has significantly impeded the development of a more comprehensive concept of psychiatric rehabilitation; third, the shrinking of available economic resources caused by social and economic changes and reductions in the size of the state's commitment to social welfare has constrained the evolution of community-based psychiatric rehabilitation programs (Chang *et al.* 2002: 32, 33).

It seems that the absence and passivity of the state and governmental institutions in taking care of mental ill persons is just accepted by the population as a reality that is difficult to change. But this conclusion has to be examined through comparing it to the way China has responded to HIV/AIDS epidemic since the late 1980s.

Engagement and Intervention: National Reaction to HIV/AIDS Epidemic

Although the Chinese government appeared to deny and ignore the HIV/AIDS epidemic until the late 1990s, it changed its attitude dramatically after the SARS crisis (2002–2003) in the early 2000s. Owing to increasing international criticism, its own desire for membership in a global world and maybe feelings of guilt by many local governmental institutions' involvement in HIV/AIDS cases caused through blood selling, the government turned to take a relatively open stance toward relevant information release and international aid. Through cooperating with WHO and many foreign organizations, the state's institutions at all levels have been involved deeply and actively with this epidemic. In 2003, the Chinese government introduced "four free and one care" policy for AIDS control, which was not only a promise but also significant embodiment of the Chinese government's engagement in fighting the HIV/AIDS epidemic. This policy, which provides free medication for AIDS patients, has been welcomed globally and is greatly appreciated among HIV/AIDS patients in China. But the question that has been neglected is what about other diseases, or what about other patients who have diseases, such as mental illness or hepatitis, rather than HIV/AIDS. Is it possible for them to get similar care or treatment in the near future? If not, why?

Zhanshan once told me that he felt lucky that he contracted AIDS rather than hepatitis B or C because free medication was only for HIV/AIDS patients in China. He often said so to comfort those patients who tested HIV positive when he was applying crisis intervention. I did not believe that he was telling the truth about how he really felt about his HIV/AIDS status, but he did reveal something important: Only HIV/AIDS patients get free medication. That fact made me think what this national policy, free medication only for the HIV/AIDS patients, is really about. Why HIV/AIDS, not other diseases? Is it because HIV/AIDS became a popular topic in the global context and attracted more and more international concern and funds? Why doesn't this policy apply to the patients with other diseases? Is it because the other diseases appeared not that dangerous to the regime as did HIV/AIDS? How would those patients with other diseases feel about this policy? I later read from the internet that many patients who had other diseases, especially serious hepatitis, complained and became angry with the logic of this policy, which sounded unreasoning to them. Essentially, these hepatitis patients argued, this policy implies that those "shameless" people (referring to people with HIV/AIDS) in their eyes even got free medication while they (hepatitis patients), who did nothing wrong, could not have it. Hepatitis is also highly stigmatized in China; none of work units or companies would hire people with active hepatitis. Apparently hepatitis patients were not just criticizing inequality caused by this policy; instead, this policy simply appeared morally wrong rather than merely unfair to hepatitis patients, whose accusation was not just that they did not get the same national policy of free medication as did HIV/AIDS patients, but that they challenged who deserved the policy of free medication. Hepatitis patients' accusation was a moral judgment and also related with the embodiment of stigma associated with HIV/AIDS.

To explain the Chinese government's active engagement in fighting the HIV/AIDS epidemic, the issue of timing has to be taken into account. A variety of factors might have combined exactly at that moment to force the state to react to the epidemic that way. However, a comparison of the national polices respectively applied to HIV/AIDS epidemic, mental illness and hepatitis tells us that the government's response is based on its own concern, rather than a coincidence. In contrast to the state's active intervention in AIDS control, mental illness and hepatitis are ignored and neglected by the state. In the eyes of the Chinese government, the danger posed by HIV/AIDS epidemic to the regime and the entire country definitely matters much more than that caused by mental illness or hepatitis. No matter that the danger brought by HIV/AIDS epidemic has been considered as an epidemic dangerous to public health, a moral danger that disgraces the country, a threat that delegitimatizes the country's membership in global world, or all of above, it really matters more. It matters because it has been perceived as a signal danger to shehui anding (societal security and stability), which has always been the first and foremost concern for Chinese government; while mental illness and hepatitis remain an individual or family problem, which is not assumed to be able to threaten societal security and stability in any serious way. Although mentally ill persons do appear as danger to public safety, this danger is assumed to remain in local communities and has never presented itself as a threat requiring collective action, such as collective shangfan and collective demonstration.[2] In a sense, HIV/AIDS epidemic constitutes a serious danger to what matters most to the state while mental illness does not, at least yet, which explains the state's relative indifference to mental illness.

In speaking of the state and governmental institutions' engagement in dealing with HIV/AIDS epidemic, the personal attitude toward HIV/AIDS among party and governmental cadres has to be taken into account. The personal attitude of the policy makers in China tells us more about the implication of national policy on AIDS control. Research (Jin 2005) conducted in Beijing in 2005 demonstrated that stigma associated with HIV/AIDS was quite common among party and governmental cadres. A sample of 380 party and governmental cadres from different provinces was drawn from those who studied at the Central Party School during 2001–2004.[3] The research result showed that, among these cadres, 34% agree that only gay men and people who visited prostitutes are likely to contract AIDS; 36% agree that only drug users are likely to contract AIDS; 36% agree to put restriction on HIV/AIDS patients' professional opportunities; 39% agree to separate HIV/AIDS patients from healthy people; 65% agree to separate members who contracted HIV/AIDS from their own families; 23% do not know what to do in that situation; 13% are willing to care for family members who contracted HIV/AIDS; 60% agree to fire subordinates who contracted HIV/AIDS; 16% agree to publish subordinate's AIDS status within work unit and then fire him/her;

---

[2] In China, governments at all levels are extremely sensitive to collective actions, which are considered serious danger to social order and societal stability. Hence, collective action is generally not allowed in the legal sense. As a rule, organizers of collective actions have to apply to and get permission from public security bureaus. Application for permission is usually considered "turning yourself in" and zitouluowang (falling into trap), which none would want to try. Ironically, people who want to appeal to higher authorities for justice have to play with this rule from time to time. Suffering or injustice fallen upon individual or family can hardly attract higher authorities' attention unless it turns to a collective action. Once it appears in the form of collective action, higher authorities have to look into it for fear that it may cause instability in the society.

[3] In China, only those party and governmental cadres who are considered having a promising future in the political system will be offered the opportunity to study at the Central Party School. Hence, studying at the Central Party School is generally a sign that the cadre is selected by higher authorities and will be elevated in the near future. Therefore, this research's results can be very helpful and valid in finding out the dominant attitude toward HIV/AIDS among the policy makers in China.

20% do not know what to do in that situation. The clear distinction between the party and governmental cadres' personal attitude to HIV/AIDS and the state's AIDS policy further suggests that Chinese government's active engagement in caring for HIV/AIDS patients is much more based on its concern about societal security and stability, rather than on a less stigmatizing attitude toward HIV/AIDS patients.

Implication of Non-Person and Non-Human: A Source of Social Insecurity

Comparison of the state's reactions and public responses between mental illness and HIV/AIDS further shows what the existence of non-persons and non-humans means to local communities and the state. For people with mental illness and HIV/AIDS, being a non-person or a non-human implies social exclusion; for local community, the existence of non-humans and non-humans implies a threat to public safety; for the state and governmental institutions, it implies a source of social insecurity, which poses a threat to societal stability.

Social exclusion implies a person has no position in the society. The person is not socially recognized or identified. In other words, non-humans and non-persons are not assumed to exist in the society, even if they do in reality. Hence, social exclusion directly leads to the absence and passivity of social institutional arrangements with respect to mental illness, which further strengthens the feeling of unsafety among local communities. As I heard time and again in field work, in the face of people with mental illness, especially psychosis, who are considered potentially violent and dangerous, many people simply replied in defending their discrimination against the mentally ill persons, "It is not that I want to discriminate against them; what I am concerned about is what if I get hurt. Who is going to be responsible for that? No one. The state does not have any shuofa about it." Shuofa is a way of saying something or a statement; the state's shuofa refers to governmental attitudes, explanations and institutional arrangements in the face of particular events. The absence of governmental shuofa in regard to mental illness leads to a common impression among the general population that people with mental illness can hurt others without being punished; likewise, people with mental illness can also be hurt without punishment.

Being non-humans or non-persons, people with mental illness are considered a serious threat to public safety within local communities, but this threat is not assumed to be dangerous enough to threaten the safety and security of the entire society, which is the reason that the state and governmental institutions tend to avoid, ignore or play a passive role in dealing with mental illness. On the contrary, HIV/AIDS epidemic has been perceived by the state as a threat to the entire society and a source of social insecurity, which results in the Chinese government's active engagement in fighting HIV/AIDS epidemic. China' "four free and one care" AIDS policy is more the embodiment of the state's concern about societal security; the policy is mainly based on the state's perception of the epidemic as a source of societal insecurity. For the state, to care or not to care depends on whether there is a threat to societal security and stability.

Qishi: The Chinese View of Discrimination

Looking back at hepatitis patients' responses to the Chinese government's AIDS control policy and the public responses to Tingting's case: Hepatitis patients criticized the policy for its moral implication: "shameless" AIDS patients get free medication while "innocent" hepatitis patients do not. Yet they seemed to have been irritated more by this morally wrong policy rather than by their own situation of being left uncared for. In Tingting' case, few people thought about the responsibility that the state through its governmental institutions should have taken in the family tragedy. The common belief that taking care of people with mental illness or hepatitis is just an individual or family duty certainly contributes to these public responses. This common belief can be rephrased as: Anyone outside of the family who does not do anything about it will not be considered irresponsible or morally problematic. To understand this point, one has to take into account what avoiding or ignoring means with respect to stigma in the Chinese context.

A Taiwanese anthropologist translated stigma into Chinese in his work (Xie 1987), in which stigma translated as wuming (stained name). In the early 2000s, the conception of stigma was introduced by international organizations into mainland China when they started participating in China' fight against the HIV/AIDS epidemic. After that, Chinese scholars started using stigma and translated it as xiuru (humiliation) (Chen *et al.* 2004; Shi *et al.* 2004) or chiru (shame) (Wang and Zhang 2006). Other scholars simply use qishi (discrimination against), and most do not use wuming (Liu 2005). The fact that it is difficult to find a Chinese counterpart of stigma suggests that stigma might have never been considered a problem in Chinese culture. Yet the meaning and practice that stigma refers to have a long history in China and can be traced back to an ancient Chinese penalty: qing. According to shuowenjiezi (an ancient Chinese dictionary, "qing, moxing zai mian ye." Qing is a penalty imposed to leave a mark on the face of criminals: brand a character or tattoo on the criminals' face, and then dye it with black ink. The mark left on the face then remains visible in public for the rest of their lives, indicating that they used to be criminals and had been punished for their misdeeds. According to *Shangjunshu — shangxing* (a document written in Shang Dynasty), qing, as a penalty, was meant to make criminals feel ashamed and prevent them from committing crimes again rather than to psychically hurt them. In this sense, China has a long history of using humiliation and shame to actualize punishment and, more importantly, social control. Under both Nationalist and Communist governments, techniques of shaming enemies were widely employed.

Qishi (discrimination against) is also seldom used in China. Qi originally refers to branching roads and generally means being extra, divergent, different, or inconsistent; shi means looking at, inspecting, or treating. Qishi did not attract much public attention until recently. It came to be related to cases in which physically disabled persons, hepatitis patients, persons with psychosis, HIV/AIDS patients, and people from particular areas in China were classified as marginalized and the objects of discrimination. For example, people from Henan province, one of China's poorest and oldest regions, have been the target of accusation of community, are discriminated against.[4] Qishi did not come to be an academic topic until it

[4] In 2005, a local police department in Shenzhen put up a poster in a neighborhood, stating "Take Henanese criminals off the streets", which soon became controversial and started up a national debate about people from Henan province. People from other provinces began accusing Henanese for being liars, cheaters, and criminals while Henanese stood up against these accusations and blamed the others for stigmatizing Henanese.

was introduced into studies of the HIV/AIDS epidemic. Among the general population, qishi is seldom used.

In the Chinese view, qishi often refers to behaving in an aggressive way toward another person, such as teasing, shouting at, spitting at, or beating others. That is to say, one has to do something aggressive to constitute qishi. Aggressive action is a necessary factor for qishi. People define qishi in terms of specific actions rather than an attitude. As I observed in field work, many people, when they were asked about qishi, often felt lost at first, and then started to list a number of aggressive actions. It suggests that qishi has to take place in the process of interpersonal interactions in a particular context. Without specific interactions happening in a particular context, there will be no qishi. None of my informants consider avoiding or ignoring others to be types of qishi because they believe that nothing has been actively done against others in that situation. Avoiding and ignoring behaviors are the most common forms of stigmatization in China, which is the reason that most of people do not consider themselves stigmatizers and refuse to admit that qishi is a serious social problem; instead, qishi is often considered an individual problem only related to some people who experience direct psychological or physical assault.

Second, qishi implies seeing and treating somebody as weak, physically, mentally or socially. That is to say, the objects of qishi have to be the weak to constitute qishi. In Chinese view, this point can be rephrased as: a person is discriminated against only because he/she is one of the weak. In general, it is widely accepted that teasing, beating, shouting or spitting at the members of the disadvantaged groups, such as the poor and physically disabled persons, is not the right thing to do and people do so out of lack of sympathy for the weak should feel ashamed. As I often found in field work, however, Chinese people are usually unwilling to admit that they are discriminated against for fear being linked to the weak and vulnerable, which makes them feel ashamed and lose face; they may describe the events, in which they are discriminated against, but they often hesitate to use the word about themselves. If the objects are persons with mental illnesses, especially psychosis, who are considered non-persons because they are not assumed to be able to feel ashamed for being treated inhumanly, people often consider it blameless and harmless to treat them as non-persons. And hence teasing and open ridicule of the mentally ill is not uncommon. If the objects are criminals, drug abusers or HIV/AIDS patients, who are considered non-persons because of assumed moral defects, discrimination against these people is often regarded as doing the right thing to bad persons. That is to say, open discrimination is viewed as a way to articulate one's moral stance and moral judgment. Hence, in the Chinese context, the moral sense qishi conveys is pointedly ambiguous: It implies lack of sympathy for the weak, doing something harmless to non-persons, or doing the right thing to non-persons. The difference depends on who the object is. The object's identity is the main determinant and precondition of qishi. It suggests that, in the Chinese view, the precondition of qishi is that the object must be considered a non-person who has already been excluded from the category of persons with face and rights and deprived of the right to be a responsible person, which is the exact reason that the person can be humiliated and treated without dignity. The identity of non-persons makes discrimination against them and stigmatization legitimate in the local world. In a sense, being a non-person is not the result but the precondition of stigmatization. In other words, loss of personhood happens before rather than after a person is stigmatized. Rather than depriving a person of his/her personhood, stigmatization signifies, confirms and strengthens the person's already existing non-person identity in public. Hence relative power in interpersonal relations through which the competent show contempt for the incompetent shows that vulnerability in social terms is crucial to stigma.

Third, qishi has to take place in public and has to be seen by others, making the objects feel humiliated, which especially applies to criminals, drug users and the HIV/AIDS patients. That is to say, qishi has to cause humiliating consequences to these objects in public in order to be effective. In the Chinese view, qishi is mainly about humiliation. For people with psychosis, simply avoiding, ignoring, or leaving them uncared for is enough to let them humiliate themselves in public. In addition, they are not assumed to be able to feel humiliated. Hence, it is harmless and blameless to discriminate against them. For HIV/AIDS patients, qishi is meant to make them realize their non-person identity and feel ashamed for it. That is also the reason that many people, medical professionals and governmental institutions insist that shame, humiliation and stigmatization are effective ways to prevent the spread of HIV/AIDS epidemic and actualize social control. And in the SARS epidemic this is thought by many to have been confirmed (Kleinman and Watson 2006).

Through the comparison between stigma related to mental illness and that related to HIV/AIDS, this chapter describes the micro process of stigmatization (from non-person to non-human in the case of mental illness; from non-human to non-person in the case of HIV/AIDS) in the local world, especially in the family. It also explores the local moral common sense (what makes a human or a person) and social values (what matters most to a family, community or society) inherent in the social logic of stigmatization as one of the more potent social forces, and examines the involvement of the state and government in stigmatization. My analysis shows that the local context and broader society are not separate from each other; instead, the moral common sense of what makes a human or a person, community or society-centered social values, and social institutional arrangements based on common sense and social values are the main factors that weave families, local communities and the broader society together and make stigma into a totalizing social phenomenon.

Chapter Six

Conclusion

Psychological and social psychological views dominated the early phase of stigma studies and continue to exert influence in the present day. Goffman (1963) defined stigma as a deeply discrediting attribute and a socially negative deviance. His view shaped how stigma was initially approached. Later on, Jones *et al.* (1984) developed a social psychological understanding of stigma and grounded stigma in the individual's interactions; Link and Phelan (2001) took the conception of power into account but turned to measure stigma as public attitude, which had a profound influence on the current phase of stigma studies. Such studies now reduce stigma to public attitude toward risk, and then measure that attitudinal variable quantitatively, while exploring the roots of stigma through attribution models;

Social historians and sociologists added a social perspective to the study of stigma. Gussow (1968, 1988) considered leprosy stigma in its changing social historical context and defined stigma as "a part of life rather than an undesired difference". Alonzo and Reynolds (1995) suggested that stigma is a social constructive/interactive phenomenon and placed stigma into "the broader society". Watts (1997) defined stigma principally as a social construction. In the field of public health, Parker and Aggleton (2003) relocated stigma into a structure framed by culture, power and difference and linked stigma to the reproduction of social difference.

Anthropologists' efforts in studying stigma can be traced back to Mary Douglas (1990), who added moral meaning to the conceptions of danger and risk emphasized by psychologists and considered stigma a "moralized danger". In social medicine and medical anthropology, Farmer (1992) pointed out that "sickness is a result of structural violence". Based on their research in Brazil, Abadia-Barrero and Castro (2006) found that "structural violence in the forms of poverty, racism, and inequalities in social status, gender, and age fuels children's experiences of stigma"; they proposed "structural violence as the framework to study stigma" (2005: 1219). Castro and Farmer (2005) stated that the current definition of stigma has not been "grounded in a broader biosocial understanding" and is "often desocialized — decontextualized from larger social processes that are both historically rooted and linked to persons and processes that are not visible to the survey researcher" (2005: 53). They proposed "structural violence as a conceptual framework for understanding AIDS-related stigma" (2005: 54). Fassin (2007) also depicted AIDS patients' illness experience in the historical and political context featuring social inequality. There is no doubt that structural violence — larger social forces-is involved in stigma, but questions remain. Is there any social suffering to which structural violence has not contributed? Then, exactly what kind of role does structural violence play in stigma? More importantly, what does it mean to be a member of disadvantaged groups in a society? If it is decontextualized to consider stigma without taking larger social forces into account, it will be decontextualized too to consider stigma without paying attention to the local world where stigma is practiced in reality against subject's agency.

Biehl (2005) described people with mental illness and HIV/AIDS in Brazil who were regarded as ex-humans living in a zone of social abandonment. Kleinman (1988) emphasized cultural meaning behind the issue of stigma, and then identified stigma as "a moral experience" (Yang *et al.* 2007). My major concern in this research is to look further into stigma by developing the definition — stigma as a moral experience — in order to explore exactly what kind of moral meaning is involved in stigma associated with mental illness and HIV/AIDS and to illustrate this by showing how stigma has been practiced with respect to illness experience in the context of China.

Stigma: A Totalizing Social Phenomenon

I would argue that structural violence is rather the embodiment than the root of stigma. Structural violence is the way stigma has been actualized in the life world. As I have described in the ethnography sections, stigma is a totalizing social phenomenon constituted, shaped, maintained and strengthened by the joint forces of government policies, institutions, cultural construction and daily moral practices in local context. Accordingly, government, work units, health care system, schools, local communities and families are all involved in the process of stigmatization. Stigma is neither a problem of the stigmatized, nor a problem of stigmatizers; instead, it is a problem of all of us rather than others — those stigmatizers. People stigmatize not because they are ignorant or morally degenerate (lack of sympathy) as is assumed by many. Stigma is about the basic moral common sense and fundamental social values on which a society is based and managed.

Stigma: Pervasive Life Experience

The reality of people with mental illness or HIV/AIDS being stigmatized does not necessarily start when they are diagnosed with mental illness or test HIV positive, as a number of cases I included show. Many patients had been stigmatized and discriminated against much earlier, before they had these diseases: they were stigmatized because of their disabilities; they were stigmatized when they quit school; they were stigmatized when they could not find jobs; they were stigmatized when their gay identity was found out; they were stigmatized when they were caught using drugs and sent to the local detox centers. Many of the patients I met in field had a long history of experience with stigma, which was not exclusively related to the two illnesses I studied in my research. More importantly, they often considered their entire life a continuum of being stigmatized rather than different phases constituted by different kinds of stigma. For them, there was no way to differentiate one stigma from another. Being stigmatized is a pervasive and endless life experience of being socially excluded and treated as non-persons. This fact suggests that mental illness and HIV/AIDS are not the only factors that can make a person into a non-person or non-human. In a sense, either mental illness or HIV/AIDS is just one of various carriers of stigma. Stigma, then, is brought to the person, carried by particular social phenomenon, which is not stigmatized itself. Hence, the key to understand stigma associated with mental illness and HIV/AIDS goes beyond the diseases themselves; instead, the key is to find out how the two diseases compromise the patients' personhood, which lies in the moral common sense concerning what makes a person in local context.

Family: A Crucial Site for Stigma

Focusing on stigmatization within the family is helpful to avoid reducing stigma into a public attitude toward certain diseases and ending up measuring so imagined stigma among the general population. Moreover, among the various sites, including the family, community, work unit, health care system and governmental institution, where stigma has been actualized in China, the family is the most crucial one. Because it is the site in which patients and their family members are engaging in the closest interactions and relationships. It is in these most intimate interpersonal relationships that the social logic of stigma and social mechanisms of stigmatization can be observed and understood.

Stigmatization: Practices of Local Moral Meaning

As my ethnographic materials showed, stigma related to either mental illness or HIV/AIS is not just the generalized public perception of health risk or public attitude toward health threat posed by these diseases; instead, it implies a strong emotion toward the patients, their families, even the local communities to which they belong, which are all judged by local moral meaning for what they have done that caused these diseases and what they have done to their families and the local communities by bringing these diseases into the privileged social spaces. This judgment directly leads to another moral judgment about the identity of the patients and their families. Hence, stigmatization is a moral response toward what really matters that has been threatened by illness experience. To stigmatize means to apply the local moral meaning to judge and punish the patients, their families, and even the local communities for what they have done that has threatened what really matters in the local world.

In the Chinese context, the moral meaning of what makes a human or person is the root of stigma related to mental illness and HIV/AIDS. The practices associated with this moral meaning at different levels, including families, local communities, institutions and government, are the social mechanism that maintains and strengthens stigma. In this sense, political economics of health, which emphasize social inequality created by structural violence, might not be able to see and explain this moral meaning. In China, the government started providing free HIV testing, medication and counseling for HIV/AIDS patients since 2003, but many patients and their family members continue to refuse to take the test or participate in counseling because of shame, even if there was no need to worry about the cost. In Dexin, some patients quit treatment apparently not because they could not afford it; some moved the entire family to other cities to hide the shame brought about by AIDS status. They had to come back to the clinic to get medication refills each month from hundreds of miles away. Stigma related to mental illness and HIV/AIDS is not just that social inequality causes patients to be unable to afford medication or quality care. Lower cost does help make medication and health care more accessible and empowers more and more patients and their families to be able to handle the critical health condition, but it does not help reduce stigma. Just imagine whether an HIV/AIDS patient would feel that he is less stigmatized just because the government gave him free medication so he could afford treatment. Apparently not. Would anyone feel that he or she should not stigmatize mentally ill persons or HIV/AIDS patients just because they have quality care? People do stigmatize the poor, but they do not stigmatize these patients just because they are too poor to afford treatment or quality care.

Social inequality has existed as a persistent social problem in every society and I believe that it will continue to be a social problem in future, given the fact that no society is and will be able to provide the same quality treatment to all marginalized and disadvantaged groups. Simply providing better treatment and quality care to a part of the marginalized population does not help resolve the stigma problem.

Moreover, it may create further social inequality and even foster and strengthen the stigma associated with particular groups. It is true that stigma has to be observed in the broader social context shaped by social inequality; but, without considering the micro processes and local context of stigma, it will be difficult to understand what stigma means to people who live with it and therefore what it is actually about. As Jackson argued, "it would be facile to reduce the meaning of a person's existence to either such external circumstances or to some inner essence" (Jackson 2005).

Non-Person: The Precondition of Stigma in the Local Context

It has been widely agreed that stigma damages the stigmatized's personhood and consequently compromises their normal identity formation, but little attention has been paid to the real process whereby stigma leads to compromised personhood or, in reverse, compromised personhood leads to stigma. I would argue that in public when people can only imagine the mentally ill persons or HIV/AIDS patients with whom they have no direct contact, stigma definitely leads to damage the patients' personhood and compromise their identities; but in the local context where people frequently engage in close interpersonal relationships with these patients, the process is the opposite: stigma comes after compromised personhood. Stigma is a result rather than the root of compromised personhood or identity. Hence, in the local context, a person is stigmatized because his or her personhood and identity has already been damaged and he or she already has become a non-person; losing personhood or identity is the very reason that the person is stigmatized. A person can only be stigmatized after he or she has been categorized into the group of non-persons.

In the case of mental illness, people often assume that the patients are unable to be a person, so they reduce them to non-persons, and stigmatize them. HIV/AIDS patients are regarded as non-persons and are stigmatized because what they had done (or it is imagined they had done) that caused their AIDS revealed that they failed to be a person.

Social Exclusion and Social Insecurity: Implication of Being a Non-Person

For people with mental illness or HIV/AIDS, being a non-person implies social exclusion, meaning that one belongs nowhere, has no rights, and possesses no protections; for families, members with such diseases imply a challenge and threat to family relationships and family values; for local communities, the existence of these patients poses a threat to public security; for the state, they constitute a threat to societal security and stability. To care or not to care about those who are afflicted depends on whether what matters most has been perceived to be seriously threatened.

Stigma: A Dynamic Social Process

I refer non-persons to people who have no social acceptance and non-humans to people who have no family acceptance. As I described in Chapter five, within the context of the family, persons with mental illness, especially psychosis, generally experience identity transformation from being a person to being a non-person and onto being a non-human (in the extreme cases) over the course of the entire family's experience of fighting the mental illness. When a person appears to have psychosis, the entire family begins to seek help (at first within family, then among relatives) and hides the patient at home. They hide the patient both to protect him or her and also protect the family from shame. Eventually they have to turn to mental hospitals for help. In the end, when the patient's psychosis becomes visible in local community, the patient is soon considered a non-person without social acceptance or status, while the patient still remains a person within the family. The family continues to take care of the patient at home. In the case of violent and uncontrollable psychosis, the family often ends up sending the patient to a mental hospital after years of family care. After one or more episodes of institutionalization, they then very likely abandon the patient. This is when the patient is considered non-human by society — an individual rejected by his/her own family without connection to or protection from family. In the most extreme case, the family is possibly forced to kill the patient because of shame and social pressure, or out of love because the family seeks to end the patient's suffering.

In the case of HIV/AIDS, patients often experience the opposite process. They go from being a person to being a non-human and onward to being a non-person over the process of the entire family's struggle to hide the shame brought about by HIV/AIDS status. Stigma related to HIV/AIDS is often associated with that related to gay identity or drug abuse. Each of these means treachery to the family in the Chinese context. Hence, once a person's HIV/AIDS status is known within the family, the person is likely to be considered a non-human by family members and blamed for what he or she did that caused HIV/AIDS and brought the shame to the entire family. But the family has to hide the HIV/AIDS status of the patient for fear that people outside of family may get to know it. The patient starts to live with a double identity: being a non-human in the family and being a person in public. For fear of the disclosure of HIV/AIDS status, the patient often has to retreat from former relationships and social networks, and then retreat further from the public sphere and, in the end, turns to live without any close relationship. By so doing, the patient makes him/herself a non-person in society. For those patients who contracted HIV/AIDS through blood transfusion or blood selling, they generally regard themselves as innocent victims and tend to speak up in public to seek help. During that process, they very likely publicly expose their HIV/AIDS status, and then they are soon considered non-persons by others in society.

The dynamic social process of stigma further reveals that people with mental illness or HIV/AIDS are stigmatized because they are assumed not to be able to be persons or have failed to be persons; their families abandoned them because the family feels passionately that what matters most to it, family relationships and values, has been seriously threatened; the local community stigmatizes the patients and their families because that which matters most to the community, public safety, has been perceived as endangered; the state's absence and passivity in taking care of mentally ill persons and being actively engaging in caring for HIV/AIDS patients suggest that what matters much more to the state is societal security and stability.

Implications of This Research

Around the world, stigma appears to be stronger where there is an absence of programs and practices concerning humanitarian ethics and human rights (UNAIDS 2005). This is true in the Chinese society where particularism is more valued than universalism and social values are centered on community and society rather than the individual. There is no cure for stigma since there is no cure for social distinction. Yet adding humanitarian ethics to moral common sense certainly can at least make fewer people suffer and make them suffer less.

In developing humanitarian ethics and spreading thinking about human rights in China, both Chinese and outsiders representing global institutions have to face a dilemma that took form during former interactions on human rights: namely, politicization of human rights. In China, both government officials and the general public tend to believe that the idea of human rights is nothing other than a weapon that western countries often use to denigrate and attack China. However, there is a change in the way the Chinese government responds to international criticism on its human rights condition. The Chinese government used to simply refuse to accept criticism and blamed western countries for China bashing. More recently, the Chinese government has turned to refute criticism by arguing that the country which criticizes China also has a poor human rights condition. Hence the Chinese government questions the other countries' qualification and right to criticize China.[1] This change of response is not just a change of defensive strategy but a more hopeful sign, suggesting that the Chinese government is starting to identify with the idea of human rights, even though it does not accept criticism of its own world. Another sign showing that the Chinese government begins to accept the idea of human rights can be found in the central government's slogan: yi ren wei ben, meaning people-oriented, or to take people as the foremost.[2] In a sense, the current broader social context in China makes it possible to talk

[1] In response to the yearly Country Reports on Human Rights Practices published by the U.S. Department of State, the State Council Information Office of the Chinese government published U.S. Human Rights Records for nine consecutive years from 1999 to 2007.

[2] In 2007, a report submitted by Chinese Communist Party to the party's 17th national conference stated that social development must be people-oriented.

about and do something about the suffering of marginalized groups, including perhaps stigma.

In this broader context, the implication of my research lies in what we can do about stigma related to mental illness and HIV/AIDS in China. Based on my understanding of the social logic and social mechanism of stigma in the Chinese context, I suggest that:

1. Legislation must be the first and foremost task to fight stigma related to mental illness and HIV/AIDS. The law may not be able to change how people perceive mentally ill persons and HIV/AIDS patients, but at least it can protect the sufferers from being treated in the worst way. Sufferers deserve at least an official category of recognition and frameworks of responses under which they can seek help and protection.

2. Government should allow and encourage volunteers to work at health care, social welfare, and humanitarian assistance institutions, such as NGOs, which work with people who have mental illness or HIV/AIDS. Although it is difficult to change public attitudes in a short time, people who are willing to contact and help these patients should be allowed to do so in a way that recognizes and protects the afflicted. Regular contacts often lead to mutual familiarity and understanding. Even though it is not expected to work in every case, over the long term it can sensitize the populous to the injustice of stigma and the disability for more humane responses. Potentially, patients can get back to normal interpersonal relationships and rebuild the connection between society and socially excluded groups. Working with mentally ill persons and HIV/AIDS patients can educate volunteers, part of the general population, and help them and more and more people to get to know marginalized groups and their suffering, which is usually concealed under the surface of society.

3. Reform is needed in the current medical system in China. I suggest setting up social medicine departments or sections in hospitals, including general hospitals, and other health care institutions at all levels. This plan applies to all hospitals and health care institutions, not just those related to mental illness and HIV/AIDS. In the current China, many people now related discrimination against people with these two illnesses to the

medical staff's poor professional ethics. They blamed doctors and nurses for not fulfilling their duty. Hence, medical professionals need to be trained and encouraged by service institutions to practice ethical care with an emphasis on comprehensive care giving. Some believe that patients have developed new service needs that are not covered by the old medical system, and agree to expand medical professionals' field of work to cover patients' illness experience rather than just the biology of diseases. I suspect that this point of view might not be realistic, even though I agree that medical professionals should realize that they are working with a person rather than just dealing with the disease. Psychologists, social workers and volunteers are expected to work in social medicine departments. In general, clinical staff members could introduce patients who need help to the social medicine department. Once the members of the social medicine department get to know the patients' problems, including any problem related to their illnesses, either they take care of these, if it is possible, or they can help the patients contact other relevant institutions or governmental institutions to seek further help. Social medicine departments within hospitals can bridge the gap between health care institutions and other governmental institutions and help build a comprehensive care system to care for patients as full persons.

4. Stigma prevention campaign has to be located in the framework of long-term public education aimed to develop the concern about humanitarian ethics and human rights among the general population. First, government and its institution must officially recognize and define stigma as a social phenomenon rather than a problem only related to epidemics that can be resolved within health care system. Second, anti-stigma campaigns in China need to go beyond the current limited focus on HIV/AIDS and link themselves to a variety of unjust human conditions, including physical disability, mental illness, hepatitis, HIV/AIDS, poverty, etc. Third, the idea of humanitarian ethics has to be brought into the center of the professional education in government and its institutions, including administration system, social welfare system and health care system, which is the only way to help the country to reach a balance between focusing on economic increase and taking care of the disadvantaged population and a balance between the concern about the society and

caring for the individual in the radically changing China. Fourth, the Chinese government must allow the disadvantaged population to organize its own self-help and assistance subgroups. Thus, on one hand, the disadvantaged individuals can rebuild and maintain their social relationships and networks in order to counteract social exclusion; on the other hand, self-help and assistance groups can make their voices heard in the society and empower themselves to seek help, rights and protection. Fifth, public education concerning humanitarian ethics must combine education in public media with that in schools, which are still the most important sites in China where the general population's moral sense and social values take form. Adding humanitarian ethics to moral common sense can gradually help the idea of human rights take form among the general population in China.

References

Abadia-Barrero, C. E. and Castro, A. (2006). Experiences of stigma and access to HAART in children and adolescents living with HIV/AIDS in Brazil. *Soc. Sci. Med.*, 62(5), 1219–1228.

Alonzo, A. A. and Reynolds, N. R. (1995). Stigma, HIV and AIDS: An exploration and elaboration of a stigma trajectory. *Soc. Sci. Med.*, 41(3), 303–315.

Anderson, A. F. *et al.* (2003). China's floating population and the potentlial for HIV transmission: A social-behavioural perspective. *AIDS Care*, 15(2), 177–185.

Biehl, J. G. (2005). *Vita: Life in a Zone of Social Abandonment*. Berkeley: University of California Press.

Cao, X. B. *et al.* (2005). Origin and embodiment of discrimination against AIDS and the reducing strategy. *Chin. J. AIDS/STD*, 11(3), 235–240.

Cao, X., Sullivan, S. G., Xu, J. and Wu, Z. (2006). Understanding HIV-related stigma and discrimination in a "blameless" population. *AIDS Educ. Prev.*, 18(6), 518–528.

Castro, A. and Farmer, P. (2005). Understanding and addressing AIDS-related stigma: From anthropological theory to clinical practice in haiti. *Am. J. Public Health*, 95(1), 53–59.

Chang, D. F., Xu,Y., Kleinman, A., and Kleinman, J. (2002). Rehabilitation of schizophrenia patients in China: The Shanghai Model. In A. Cohen, A. Kleinman, and B. Saraceno (Eds.), *The World Mental Health Casebook*. New York: Kluwer, pp. 27–50.

Chen, Y. C. *et al.* (2004) Research progress on humiliation and discrimination against AIDS. *Chin. J. AIDS/STD*, 10(6), 477–478.

Chinese Ministry of Health and UNAIDS (2004). A joint assessment of HIV/AIDS prevention, treatment and care in China, December, 2003. Available on: http://data.unaids.org/una-docs/china_joint_assessment_2003_en.pdf.

Corrigan, P. W. (2007). How clinical diagnosis might exacerbate the stigma of mental illness. *Social Work*, 52(1), 31–39.

Deng, R., Li, J., Sringernyuang, L. and Zhang, K. (2007). Drug abuse, HIV/AIDS and stigmatisation in a Dai community in Yunnan, China. *Soc. Sci. Med.*, 64(8), 1560–1571.

Douglas, M. (1994) *Risk and Blame: Essays in Cultural Theory*. London and New York: Routledge.

Erving, G. (1963). *Stigma: Notes on the Management of the Spoiled Identity.* Original American edition published by Prentice-Hall Inc., Englewood Cliffs, New Jersey, USA.

Farmer, P. (1992). *AIDS and Accusation: Haiti and the Geography of Blame, Comparative Studies of Health Systems and Medical Care*. Berkeley: University of California Press.

Fassin, D. (2007). *When Bodies Remember: Experiences and Politics of Aids in South Africa, California Series in Public Anthropology*. Berkeley: University of California Press.

Feldman, M. D., Zhang, J. and Cummings, S. R. (1999). Chinese and U.S. internists adhere to different ethical standards. *J. Gen. Intern. Med.*, 14(8), 469–473.

Feng, L. and Li, Y. (2007). Speculations on some issues in drug control behavioral intervention by public security organs applied in HIV/AIDS prevention affairs. *Yunnan jingguan xueyuan xuebao* [*Journal of Yunnan Police Officer Academy*] 2, 54–56.

Gao, J. *et al.* (2004). Survey on HIV/AIDS-related stigma and discrimination among residents in a rural community with a past history of paid blood donation. *Zhongguo aizibing xingbing* [*Chin. J. AIDS & STD*] 10(3), 175–177.

Goffman, E. (1963). *Stigma; Notes on the Management of Spoiled Identity, a Spectrum Book*. Englewood Cliffs, N. J.: Prentice-Hall.

Gussow, Z. (1989). *Leprosy, Racism, and Public Health: Social Policy in Chronic Disease Control*. Boulder: Westview Press.

Heller, P. S. (1973). The strategy of health sector planning. In M. Wegman, T. Lin and E. F. Purcell (Eds.), *Public health in People's Republic of China*. New York: Josiah Macy Jr Foundation.

Hesketh, T., Li, L., Ye, X., Wang, H., Jiang, M. and Tomkins, A. (2006). HIV and syphilis in migrant workers in eastern China. *Sex. Transm. Infect.* 82(1), 11–14.

Hou, Y. G., MunaiReha, and Chen, G. (2004). A way to participate in the precaution and treatment of STD/AIDS for the groups being inferior position. *Journal of the Central University for Nationalities* (Philosophy and Social Sciences Edition), 31(3), 52–57.

Huang, L. H. *et al.* (2006). Epidemiological analysis of AIDS in Dali prefecture in 2004. *Jibing Jiance [Disease Surveillance]*, 21(3), 130–132.

Jackson, M. (2005). *Existential Anthropology: Events, Exigencies, and Effects.* New York: Berghahn Books.

Jiarimuji, (2007), On the Liangshan Yi's Traditional Practice of Hospice Care. (Chinese article online) http://www.face21cn.cn/renleixue/yanjiu/article_2007_12_14_1440.html.

Jin, H., Hampton Atkinson, J., Yu, X., Heaton, R. K., Shi, C., Marcotte, T. P., Young, C., Sadek, J., Wu, Z. and Grant, I. (2006). Depression and suicidexinty in HIV/AIDS in China. *J. Affect Disord.*, 94(1–3), 269–275.

Jin, W. (2005). Analysis of the finding of a survey regarding discrimination against HIV/ AIDS among government and Party officials. *Chin. J. AIDS/STD*, 11(2), 88–90.

Jing J. (2006). The Social Origins of AIDS Panics in China. In *AIDS and Social Policy in China*, J. Kaufman, A. Kleinman, and T. Saich (Eds.). Cambridge, MA: HIV/AIDS Public Policy Project, Kennedy School of Government, Harvard University, pp. 152–169.

Jones, E. E. *et al.* (1984). *Social Stigma: The Psychology of Marked Relationships.* New York: W.H. Freeman.

Kleinman, A. (1988). *The Illness Narratives: Suffering, Healing, and the Human Condition.* New York: Basic Books.

Kleinman, A. (2006). *What Really Matters: Living a Moral Life Amidst Uncertainty and Danger.* Oxford, New York: Oxford University Press.

Kleinman, A. and Watson, J. L. (2006). *SARS in China: Prelude to Pandemic?* Stanford, CA: Stanford University Press.

Kleinman, A. and Lin, T.-Y. (1981). *Normal and Abnormal Behavior in Chinese Culture.* Dordrecht, Boston: D. Reidel; Hingham, MA: Kluwer Boston.

Kohrman, M. (1999). Grooming "que zi": Marriage exclusion and identity formation among disabled men in contemporary China. *American Ethnologist*, 26(4), 890–909.

Li, L., Wu, Z., Zhao, Y., Lin, C., Detels, R. and Wu, S. (2007). Using case vignettes to measure HIV-related stigma among health professionals in China. *Int. J. Epidemiol.*, 36(1), 178–184.

Link, B. G. and Phelan, J. C. (2001). Conceptualizing stigma. *Annual Review of Sociology*, 27, 363–385.

Link, B. G., Yang, L. H., Phelan, J. C. and Collins, P. Y. (2004). Measuring mental illness stigma. *Schizophr. Bull.*, 30(3), 511–541.

Lin, T. Y. (1985). The shaping of Chinese psychiatry in the context of politics and public health. In Lin, T. Y. and Eisenberg, L. (Eds.), *Mental Health Planning for One Billion People*. Vancouver: University of British Colombia Press.

Liu, H., Hu, Z., Li, X., Stanton, B., Naar-King, S. and Yang, H. (2006). Understanding interrelationships among HIV-related stigma, concern about HIV infection, and intent to disclose HIV serostatus: A pretest-posttest study in a rural area of eastern China. *AIDS Patient Care STDS*, 20(2), 133–142.

Liu, N. (2005). HIV AIDS, stigma, and social discrimination: A quantitative analysis of aids patients and ordinary villagers in two Chinese rural communities. *Sociological Research*, 6, 136–164.

Mann, J. (1987). Statement at an informal briefing on AIDS to the 42nd Session of the United Nations General Assembly, 20 October, New York.

Marshall, G. (1998). *Oxford Dictionary of Sociology*. Oxford and New York: Oxford University Press.

National Intelligence Council (2002). The next wave of HIV/AIDS: Nigeria, Ethiopia, Russia, India, China. ICA 2002-04 D. Available on: http://www.fas.org/irp/nic/hiv-aids.html.

Parker, R. and Aggleton, P. (2003). HIV and AIDS-related stigma and discrimination: a conceptual framework and implications for action. *Soc. Sci. Med.*, 57(1), 13–24.

Pearson, V. (1995). *Mental Health Care in China: State Policies, Professional Services and Family Responsibilities*. London; Gaskell; New York: American Psychiatric Press.

Peng, Z. *et al.* (2006). Knowledge, Attitudes, and Practice about HIV/AIDS of Public Health Professionals in Some Areas of China. *Zhongguo yaowu yilaixing zazhi* [*Chin. J. Drug Dependence*] 15(1), 49–52.

Rummel, R. J. (1991). *China's Bloody Century: Genocide and Mass Murder since 1900*. New Brunswick: Transaction Publisher.

Shi, X. M. and Zheng, X. W. (2004). Humiliation and discrimination against HIV/AIDS. *Chin J. AIDS/STD*, 10(1), 67–75.

Tang, Y. *et al.* (2004). An Investigation on Knowledge and Attitude of AIDS among Rural Residents. *Shiyong yufang yixue* [*Practical Preventive Medicine*] 11(2), 266–268.

Volinn, I. J. (1989). Issues of definitions and their implications: AIDS and leprosy. *Soc. Sci. Med.*, 29(10), 1157–1162.

Walkey, F. H., Taylor, A. J. W. and Green, D. E. (1990). Attitudes to AIDS: A comparative analysis of a new and negative stereotype. *Social Science & Medicine*, 30(5), 549–552.

Wang, F. (2008). Analysis on the factors influencing attitudes and practices related to HIV/AIDS discrimination among rural inhabitants. *Zhongguo jiankang jiaoyu* [*Chinese Journal of Health Education*] 24(8), 569–571.

Watts, S. (1997). *Epidemics and History: Disease, Power and Imperialism*. New Haven: Yale University Press.

Wang,Y. and Zhang, K. (2006). HIV/AIDS stigma and discrimination in health care services. *Shengzhi yixue zazhi* [*J. Reprod. Med.*] 15(1), 67–70.

Wang, Y., Zhang, Y., Yang, Y. *et al.* (2002). Evaluvation of the work for non-discrimination against people living with HIV and AIDS in rural area. *Zhongguo Xingbing Alizibing Fangzhi* [*Chinese Journal of STD & AIDS Prevention Control*], 8(6), 343–345.

Ware, N. C., Wyatt, M. A. and Tugenberg, T. (2005). Adherence, stereotyping and unequal HIV treatment for active users of illegal drugs. *Soc. Sci. Med.*, 61(3), 565–576.

Wu, Z., Rou, K., Xu, C. Lou, W. and Detels, R. (2005). Acceptability of HIV/AIDS counseling and testing among premarital couples in China. *AIDS Educ. Prev.*, 17(1), 12–21.

Xie, S. (1987). *Stigmatized Identity: Ethnic Change of Taiwan Aborigines*. Taipei: The Independence Evening Post.

Yan, Y. (1996). *The Flow of Gifts: Reciprocity and Social Networks in a Chinese Village*. Stanford, California: Stanford University Press.

Yang, H., Li, X., Stanton, B. Fang, X. Lin, D. and Naar-King, S. (2006). HIV-related knowledge, stigma, and willingness to disclose: A mediation analysis. *AIDS Care*, 18(7), 717–724.

Yang, L. H., Kleinman, A., Link, B. G., Phelan, J. C., Lee, S. and Good. B. (2007) Culture and stigma: Adding moral experience to stigma theory. *Soc. Sci. Med.*, 64(7), 1524–1535.

Yin, D. K. (2000). The current situation, problem and strategy of Chinese mental health work: Report on China/WHO awareness raising symposium. *Chinese Mental Health Journal*, 14(1), 4–5.

Zhang, M. Y. (2006). Challenge to mental health service in China: Thinking from world mental health surveys. *J. Shanghai Jiaotong Univ.* (*Medical Science*), 26(4), 329–334.

Zhou, R. J. and Cao, D. J. (2004). Opinions of Experts: Eliminating bias in order to help recovered people with mental illnesses to return to society. (Article on Xinhua website) http://news.xinhuanet.com/newscenter/2004-10/10/content_2072126.htm.

Zhou, Y. R. (2007). "If you get AIDS... you have to endure it alone": Understanding the social constructions of HIV/AIDS in China. *Soc. Sci. Med.*, 65(2), 284–295.

Index

CPSIA information can be obtained at www.ICGtesting.com
Printed in the USA
BVOW06*1421120216

436507BV00001B/2/P

9 781938 134807